Meals Without Squeals

Child Care
Feeding Guide and Cookbook

Christine Berman, MPH, RD
and
Jacki Fromer

Bull Publishing Company
Palo Alto, California

Bull Publishing Company
P.O. Box 208
Palo Alto, California 94302-0208
(415) 322-2855

ISBN 0-923521-10-0

Distributed in the U.S. by:
Publishers Group West
4065 Hollis Street
Emeryville, CA 94608

**Library of Congress
Cataloging-in-Publication Data**
Berman, Christine.
     Meals without squeals : child care feeding guide and cookbook /
by Christine Berman, Jacki Fromer.
                p.   cm.
     Includes bibliographical references and index.
     ISBN 0-923521-10-1 : $14.95
     1. Children—Nutrition.   2. Cookery.   I. Fromer, Jacki.
II. Title.
TX361-C5B47   1991
649'.3—dc20   91-4998
                                                   CIP

Cover Design: Robb Pawlak
Cover Photographer: Barry Shapiro
Interior Design: Maura McAndrew
Production Manager: Helen O'Donnell
Compositor: The Cowans
Display and Text Face: Palatino
Printer: Delta Lithograph Co.

First printing: July 1991

TO OUR CHILDREN

**Wynter and Mai
Reed and Rachel**

Acknowledgements

Special thanks to Carol Larson for generosity of time and computer expertise in spite of an incredibly busy schedule, Reed Fromer and Peter White for guidance in editing and organizing, and David Fromer for artistry, and those invaluable, enthusiastic pep talks.

And with loving appreciation—

To our family members for their assistance, encouragement, confidence, suggestions, patience and love—David, Reed and Rachel Fromer, Mitch Berman, Wynter and Mai Grant, Carol, Brad, Matthew and Sierra Larson, Ann Spake and Jon Fromer.

To our dear friends and associates for their ideas, critiques, generosity, enthusiasm, moral support, friendship and recipes — Barbara Abrams, DRPH, RD; Rita Abrams; Charlotte Albert; Pat Ayotte; Katy Baer, MPH, RD; Nina Baker; Judy Bartlett; Linda Bartshire; Elaine Belle; Georgia Berry; Ruth Bramell; Marek Cepietz; Doris Disbrow, DRPH, RD; Doris Fredericks, MED, RD; Elazar Freidman; Diana Goodrow; Robin Goodrow and Vanilla; Gail Hartman; Geri Henchy, MPH, RD; Bev Hoffman; Paula James; Sally Jones; Steven Kipperman; Mallory and Kevin Kopple; DeLona Kurtz; Sharon and Chiya Landry; Belinda Laucke; the staff of Marin Head Start; Elizabeth McGrady; Anne Milkie; Hannah Moore; Eileen Nelson; Katie O'Neill, MPH, RD; Lloyd Partch; Bayla Penman; Karen Jeffrey Pertschuk, MPH, RD; Johanne Quinlan; Helen Rossini; Zak Sabry, PHD; Ellyn Satter, RD, ACSW; Max Shapiro; Jackie Shonerd; Steve Susskind; Mary Syracuse; The Earth Store; Barbara Taylor; Steve Thompson; Kate Warin; Rona Weintraub; Peter White; Barbara Zeavin; Jill Zwicky, and the Marin Child Care Council staff members: Emilie Albertoli, Lynne Arceneaux, Terry DeMartini, Teresa Leibert, Mary Moore, Susan Sanders, and Hilda Castillo Wilson.

To the wonderful people at Bull Publishing for the opportunity to bring our project to fruition.

In loving memory and admiration of Florence Raskin, Katherine Fromer and Necia "Ida" Fromer.

And for the continuing inspiration we receive from child care providers and teachers who are dedicated to the well-being of children.

Contents

Foreword by Ellyn Satter

What the authors help you do couldn't be more important. Not only does good feeding allow children to eat well, but thoughtful and well-conducted meal and snack times contribute fundamentally to helping children feel secure and cared about in their child care setting.

A View from the Outside

Berman and Fromer have provided you with a wonderful book, packed full of to-the-point information and advice on preparing food and feeding children. I am going to add to what they say, but it is not because they missed it. What I have to offer is a view from the outside.

When you are in the middle of a situation, you can't always see what is going on. What I have to offer to their careful review comes from the position of the onlooker and advisor.

Parents, teachers and food program nutritionists bring their difficult feeding problems to me and I try to help them with solutions. To get so I can help, I generally go to the child care setting and observe what actually happens during eating times—as well as before and after.

I have something to add because I know what works in other settings and because I can step back from the situation and observe. No matter how good you are, if you are in the middle of dealing with something, it is hard to see what is going on.

I think all of us in our work with children could benefit from friendly observers. One person to turn to for help is a consultant with the USDA Child and Adult Care Food Program (CACFP).

As with other programs that provide reimbursement to care providers, the consultants' primary role is to review record keeping. She can also take on the role of advising and problem-solving with feeding dynamics. I know that many are not ready to tackle feeding problems. But I have worked with consultants who are, and they and their child care providers find it satisfying and helpful.

From my own role as advisor and problem-solver, here are my general observations about what distinguished the effective feeding programs.

Meals and Snacks Are an Important Part of the Program Day

One child care center I observed on behalf of a very finicky child was noisy and chaotic. Teachers served the children cafeteria style and kept on the move giving them seconds. They often didn't get to eat, themselves. None of the children ate well, but some were more compliant than my finicky little patient. Teachers encouraged and even forced the children to eat because they noticed they got cranky when they were hungry. Children were excused when they finished eating, to go to play in the gym area in the same room.

It got on my nerves to be in the midst of all that racket and hubbub, and I was not surprised at the children's poor eating. The administrator explained the rush and chaos by saying she felt a time crunch to get the children fed and leave time for their programmed activities. She hadn't realized that eating could be treated as a programmed activity.

The Teachers Sat Down with the Children to Eat

Helping another finicky three-year-old took me into her child care center to see what was happening. Children finished their morning activities with room to spare for quiet time before they ate. They sat nicely at little round tables and the room was calm and orderly while they ate.

But, instead of sitting down to eat with them, teachers took the time to put the cots out for naps. Then they took their plates and sat to eat at a table separate from the children. What happened then startled me. Every single child at every table in the room **turned to face the teachers,** and continued to face them through the rest of the meal.

Those children really wanted to know where their teachers were, and depended on making some connection with them while they ate. The feeding principle illustrated here is that children always do better with eating when someone they trust is with them.

The Food Was Nutritious and Appealing

The providers who gave their children appealing food were the ones who enjoyed eating and feeding. Some food providers spent hours in the kitchen, turning out wonderful, beautiful food that made my mouth water. Others were more pragmatic about it, used short cuts and clearly put their priorities elsewhere. But they still turned out food that was appealing, and they and the children obviously enjoyed eating it. Others seemed to feel that feeding the children was just another chore, and an unpleasant one at that. The food was drab and uninteresting and children didn't take much joy from what they were eating.

All of the providers applied nutrition principles; it was their attitude that made all the difference. To feed children well, you have to like to eat. If you don't like to eat, then someone else needs to take charge of that part of the program.

The Teachers Trusted Children to Do Their Part with Eating

Leanne Birch, a child psychologist who studies children and their eating, has demonstrated in her research that children are generally wary of new foods, but will get used to them after a while, taste them a few times (or quite a few times) and, in most cases, learn to like them. She says children learn from other children to accept new foods. And she gives us the principle of the-trusted-adult that I talked about above. All this happens, that is, unless adults get pushy and try to force or entice children to eat. Then they are less likely to eat well.

None of us would intentionally do anything that would hurt a child, but we all have our hangups about eating, and sometimes we hurt without realizing it. A friend who happens to work with child feeding programs told of her stress as she worked to get her son adjusted to a new child care setting. Part of the problem was his eating. He simply stopped eating at the child care center. He would eat an enormous breakfast and be absolutely famished when she picked him up in the afternoon. But he would not eat at school.

She could not figure it out; this was not like him. She asked the teachers and administrator if they were putting pressure on him to eat, and they reassured her they were NOT. But the problem persisted. Finally, she asked the right questions, and had her explanation.

It turned out that the policy was to not make children take food on their plates—but once they had it on their plate, the HAD to eat it. Her son's solution to that rule was simply not to take anything on his plate.

Once the problem was isolated, the teachers were amenable to changing the way they operated. They had gotten stuck on this old eating rule, and hadn't had occasion to reevaluate it.

The Teachers Were Willing to Try Out Different Approaches to Try to Help the Children

I have been amazed at what a good child care setting can accomplish with feeding, even when parents don't change the way they operate. A Child Care Food Program coordinator asked me for advice about a severe food-foraging problem they were having with a three-year-old boy. The child begged for food constantly, raided the cupboards and the refrigerator, grabbed food from the other children, and demanded second and third helpings at every meal.

The home situation was chaotic, meals were unreliable, and when the parents did feed, they restricted. They saw their son's eating as compulsive, and said they were afraid he would get too fat.

In my view, the family required a social services referral, but that option simply wasn't available. I wasn't sure anything could be done, but the child care worker wanted to give it a try, so I worked with her. (I continue to be astonished at how often the nutrition people are the only ones who are available to help child care providers.)

I told her I thought the boy needed reassurance that he was going to get enough to eat. I thought he was so food preoccupied because he was afraid he'd have to go hungry. I advised her to give the boy regular meals and snacks and to tell him repeatedly that he could have as much food as he wanted.

Between times, she was to be very firm with him that he could not panhandle for food. But she should reassure him each time she refused him a handout that another meal or snack was coming soon, and he could again have as much as he wanted.

It worked! After about three weeks of eating a lot and having tantrums over not being allowed to panhandle, the little boy's eating settled down to that of the normal toddler. The situation at home remained the same.

The Child Care Providers Knew How to Set Limits, But Also Allowed Children to be Children

Children's eating is sporadic. They pick and choose from what's available and are likely to eat only one or two food items. They accept today what they rejected yesterday, and vice versa. They eat a lot one day, and a little the next.

They automatically eat a variety, and over the space of a week or two, do meet their nutritional needs. Teachers who know this do their part by providing them with a variety of nutritious foods, but don't short order cook for them or try to force them to eat.

The Teachers Were Willing and Able to Deal Directly with Parents About Differences in Approaches to Feeding

One home child care provider talked with her parents about her feeding policies. She told them she provided children with good food, but that she did not try to control what and how much they ate.

That preparation came in handy when one day she saw her children encouraging one little girl to eat. She asked them why they were doing that. She was horrified when they told her that the little girl's father had spanked her after child care the evening before when his daughter told him she hadn't eaten all her lunch. The child care provider talked with the father, reminded him of her policies, and he stopped his pressure tactics.

In Summary, Child Care Providers Observe a Division of Responsibility in Feeding

My basic principle of feeding is this: Parents, and care providers, are responsible for *what*, *when* and *where*. Children are responsible for *how much* and *whether*. Caring adults have the primary responsibility for choosing nutritious food, for maintaining the structure of meals and snacks and for making those times pleasant. Children have the responsibility of deciding how much—and even whether—they will eat.

Throughout *Meals Without Squeals*, Berman and Fromer have demonstrated their wonderful and caring attitudes toward children and providing food for children. Feeding is more than getting food on the table. It is the whole nurturing environment that the child care provider sets up around food.

Ellyn Satter
May 1991

A Note to Parents. . .

When we fantasized about writing this book years ago, we envisioned a guidebook that child care providers and schools could use in planning their nutrition programs. But as we got to work, and the project grew, we found ourselves saying "It sure would have been nice to have this book when **our** kids were little!"

As you look through this book, you will find that some of the topics we discuss are primarily of concern to people who take care of other people's children. But we think you'll discover that most of the information we give has as much application to your home as to a child care setting. You'll also learn how to work in partnership with caregivers and teachers to make sure that children get the good nutrition they deserve.

So parents, this book is for you, too. Now, if only it had been around when **our** kids were little. . .

How To Use This Book

Meals Without Squeals is not the sort of book you must read cover-to-cover, like a novel. We wanted you to have a good place to find easily accessible answers to your questions about food and children, so we tried to address very specific topics, most in a page or two.

We suggest that you start by reading the first chapter, *What You Should Know About Feeding Children*, because that will introduce you to our philosophy and give you an overview of the important issues that come up when you are feeding children. Then look over the Table of Contents and make up your "reading list" from the subject headings that appear useful to you. Briefly, here's what you will find in *Meals Without Squeals*:

We hope you will use this book with its companion volume, *Teaching Children About Food*, because they really do complement each other. The foods that you serve and the way that you handle mealtimes are a very big part of the learning children receive about food. And a program of nutrition education can help children accept more readily the wonderful and healthful foods they're being served. Dig in and enjoy!

PART ONE

Feeding and Children

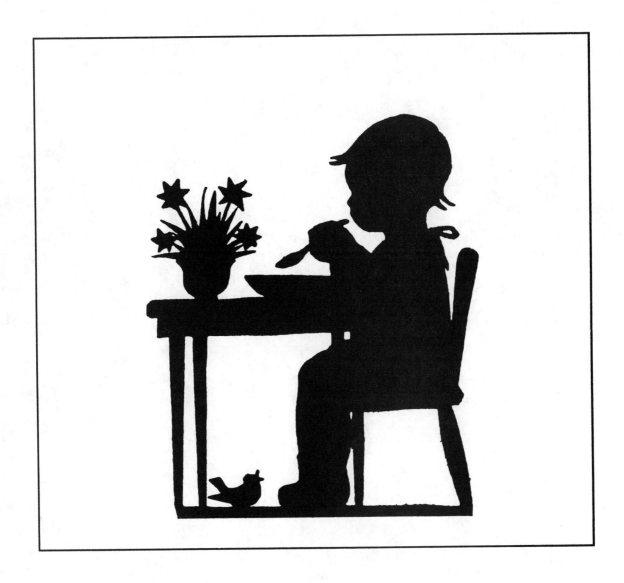

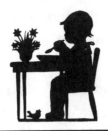

CHAPTER ONE

What You Should Know About Feeding Children

Why a Child Feeding Guide?

There are many factors that determine whether we'll enjoy long and healthy lives. Some we don't have much control over, like our heredity and our environment. Others we can do something about, such as eating habits, exercise, how we manage stress, and not smoking, drinking to excess, or using drugs. Children are in a particularly vulnerable position regarding these "lifestyle" factors. They are dependent upon adults to provide what they need in order to grow and be healthy, and they are looking to adults as role models in shaping their behaviors. We think that everyone who works with children, be they parents or caregivers, should be aware of the important connection between nutrition and children's health:

- ❏ Children need to consume the right amounts and kinds of nutrients in order to grow well, avoid overweight, tooth decay, and other problems, and to have good resistance to illness.

- ❏ Children who aren't well-nourished tend to have more problems in school. They are likely to be tired, inattentive, less curious, and less independent than their well-fed peers. They may also be irritable, less sociable, and in general have more behavior problems.[1]

❏ Eating patterns and attitudes develop during childhood that may affect health later on. More than two-thirds of the deaths in the United States are caused by diseases that can be related to eating habits: heart disease, some cancers, hypertension, and diabetes.[2]

❏ The way feeding is handled affects a child's perceptions of what to expect from the world . . . whether he will see it as a friendly and nurturing place or as a cold and frustrating one.[3]

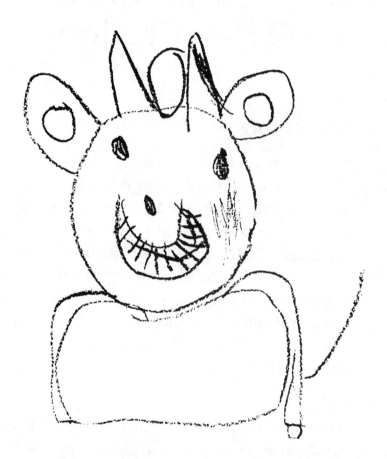

We have noticed that there is a lot of confusion among parents and caregivers about what to feed children, how to feed children, and how to teach children what they need to know in order to be healthy and happy adults. So we wrote this book to make practical information about nutrition available to anyone involved in the care of children.

The Role of the Caregiver in Children's Nutrition

It's 6 P.M. on Wednesday evening. Father has just arrived home from the office. Mother is in the kitchen putting the finishing touches on the evening meal. The cinnamony smell of fresh-baked apple pie permeates the air. Andy and Beth have just finished setting the table. Everyone washes up and sits down to a leisurely family meal. The phone does not ring, for everyone knows it's suppertime. The TV will not be turned on until the table has been cleared.

Sound familiar? Of course not! This scene is likely to be viewed on reruns of a 1960 family sitcom, but is not so typical in a real-life household of today. In fact, a recent survey of American eating habits suggests that if current domestic trends continue, the family meal could be extinct by the year 2000.[4]

In our changing society the responsibility for seeing that children are well-fed is more and more often shifting from mother-in-her-traditional-role-as-homemaker to other caregivers. Whether meals and snacks are made on site or brought from home, providers of child care have the opportunity to make a positive contribution to the nutritional well-being of children, and to offer assistance to their parents in several ways. These include:

- ❑ helping children feel good about food and eating
- ❑ helping children learn to enjoy and value healthful foods
- ❑ protecting children from such hazards as choking on food, food poisoning, and kitchen accidents
- ❑ establishing feeding policies that respect the beliefs and desires of the parents
- ❑ providing information to parents interested in improving the eating habits of their families
- ❑ keeping parents informed about their children's eating behaviors and alerting them to nutrition related problems that may require professional consultation

<u>How</u> You Feed Is As Important As <u>What</u> You Feed

You will find that we spend as much time talking about the "hows" of feeding as we do with the "whats." This is because we feel that a lot of unhappiness regarding the whole issue of food can be prevented by helping children develop a healthy relationship with food, right from the start.

Look at your own feelings about food. Do you feel like you must finish everything on your plate even if you're full already? Do you feel vague pangs of guilt about getting great enjoyment out of eating? Do you find yourself dreading having to eat? These feelings started somewhere, and for most people their origins are in childhood.

Food figures prominently in our lives from day one on, so it's important to feel positive about it and to use it appropriately. Additionally, conflicts over food can do great damage to your relationship with a child, and that's the last thing you want![5]

Ellyn Satter, in her wonderful books *Child of Mine* and *How to Get Your Kid to Eat . . . But Not Too Much*, describes the "division of responsibility in feeding"* that is central to establishing healthy feelings toward eating. Engrave this on your brain right now! It is one of the most important concepts you will ever learn.

Parents (and caregivers) are responsible for what is presented to eat and the manner in which it is presented

❑

Children are responsible for how much and even whether they eat

---

*Source: Satter, Ellyn. *How to Get Your Kid to Eat . . . But Not Too Much*. Palo Alto: Bull Publishing, 1988.

The idea that you don't have to force-feed a finicky eater, or restrain a heavy eater may be shocking at first, but it works.

Now, don't get the idea that we're advocating letting children eat *whatever* they want. Contrary to an old belief, children will not intuitively eat what is good for them, given the choice between a plate of gooey donuts and a raw vegetable platter.

(The idea that they might was a misinterpretation of some experiments a woman named Clara Davis performed in the 1930s. She confined several orphaned children to a hospital ward for long periods of time and found that they all grew beautifully when allowed to eat as much as they wanted of the foods offered to them, even when they didn't appear to be consuming a "balanced diet." The hitch is, the foods the children were offered were all natural, nutrient-dense foods like plain meats, organ meats, eggs, milk, whole grains, vegetables, fruit, and bone marrow . . . no heavily sweetened cereals, cookies, or soda pop in sight. Even Miss Davis emphasized the importance of offering nutritious, natural foods to children.)[6]

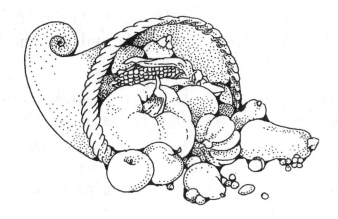

Of course, you will want to take into consideration the food preferences of your children when planning your menus, but it will be up to you to determine exactly *what* the choices will be and *when* they will be offered. The idea is to set it up so that no matter what a child eats from your offerings, he can't go wrong. Then you've done your job, and you can let the children take it from there.[7] Depending upon their age or level of development, you may have to help children with their eating. We'll talk about age-specific issues in their appropriate sections later on.

Why We Eat As We Do

Here's a little exercise for you. List three foods that you feel like eating when you're sick, or unhappy, and in need of some comforting:

_____ _____ _____

Now list three foods that you like to eat when you're celebrating a holiday or some special event:

_____ _____ _____

Last, list three foods you think of as so yukky that you can't imagine how anyone could like them:

_____ _____ _____

You see, we don't eat just to satisfy our bodies' needs for energy and growth. There are many reasons why adults and children eat, or don't eat, certain foods:

hunger	medical restrictions
taste	allergies
culture	peer pressure
habit	stress
smell	convenience
visual appeal	age
perceived nutritive value	ability to chew
to convey status	advertising
religion	previous experience
availability	seasonality
cooking ability	cravings
budget	and more . . .

What Every Child Should Learn About Food and Eating

❏ When he is hungry, that need will be met.

❏ His own food preferences will be respected.

❏ Eating is an enjoyable activity.

❏ There are ways to deal with uncomfortable feelings, besides eating.

❏ People in different cultures, and families within those cultures, have different ways of eating and different ways of celebrating special occasions with food.

❏ Our food choices affect our well-being.

❏ Food is made available through the efforts of many members of the community.

❏ In order to eat we use up resources, and we create waste that needs to be dealt with responsibly.

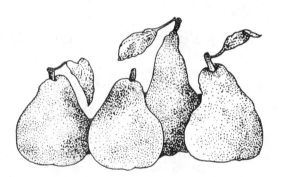

The first four concepts are crucial in the development of a child's emotional relationship with food, and the last four in his physical and social relationship with food. Review them often—together they comprise the framework for all of the discussions of child feeding and nutrition education in this book.

Children will learn these very important concepts from **you.** How you handle feeding them, how they see you relate to food and eating, the exposure you give them to the world's diversity of food habits, how you dispose of food packaging . . . all will send messages loud and clear to impressionable young minds.

Children learn that their hunger needs will be met when:

- ❑ you feed infants "on demand"
- ❑ you set up regular meal and snack times for the older children
- ❑ you help their families find resources for food, if they're having problems with it

Children learn their food preferences will be respected when:

- ❑ you let them choose what and how much to eat of what you've offered
- ❑ you ask them what they'd like when you're planning your menus

Children learn that eating is enjoyable when:

- ❑ you make sure that the mealtime environment is pleasant
- ❑ you enforce a code of behavior at the table
- ❑ you make an effort to serve foods they enjoy
- ❑ they see you enjoying eating

Children learn to deal with feelings in other ways besides overeating when:

- ❑ you encourage them to verbalize their feelings
- ❑ you resist the temptation to comfort them with cookies or candy
- ❑ they don't see you running to the cooky jar when *you're* upset

Children learn to appreciate the foodways of other cultures when:

- ❑ you plan meals that have cultural diversity
- ❑ you ask parents to contribute recipes from their own heritage or have potluck dinners with each family contributing a dish that relates to their background
- ❑ you have books and posters that show how people in other cultures eat

Children learn that our food choices affect our well-being when:

- ❑ they see you eating with the intention of providing proper nourishment for your body and you describe to them the benefits of good nutrition

Children learn about the people who provide food for them when:

- ❑ they go on field trips to markets, farms, dairies, bakeries
- ❑ they spend time in home, child care, or school kitchens

Children learn to be responsible consumers when:

- ❑ they see you making an effort to cut down on waste (food or packaging)
- ❑ they participate in gardening and get a feel for the energy that's expended to produce food
- ❑ they help with recycling projects

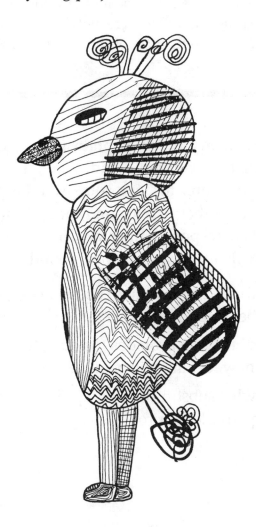

Establishing a Nutrition Philosophy Statement and Related Policies for Your Setting

We urge you to spend some time considering what you feel about the importance of nutrition for children and what your commitment to it will be in your program. You may want to do this in a group, with interested parents or staffpersons. When you are done, you should have a *nutrition philosophy statement* unique and relevant to your setting. Here's an example of what one might look like:

> We believe that good nutrition is a basic right of every child. Our nutrition policies reflect our commitment to ensuring that the children's nutritional needs will be met in a positive, nurturing manner with respect for individual needs and preferences of the children and their families.

Once you have settled on a nutrition philosphy, you have a guide that will help you determine how you will handle food and nutrition issues. Next you will find it very useful to have some written policies as well. These policies will make sure that parents and/or staff members know what to expect, or what their responsibilities are, in certain situations related to nutrition. There are many such situations, including:

- ❑ **meal schedules and routines** (who will eat with the children, what will be done about reluctant or slow eaters)
- ❑ **infant feeding** (who provides formula, how breastmilk will be stored, how feeding will be done and by whom)
- ❑ **allergies** (what substitutions will be made, whether families will be responsible for providing special foods)

- ❏ **"personal" foods** (foods brought from home, whether they are allowed, restrictions as to type)
- ❏ **celebrations** (whether you will have candy at Halloween, sweets for birthday parties)

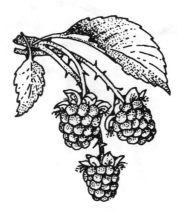

Here is an example of a child care program policy regarding foods brought from home, shared with us by the staff of the San Anselmo Preschool and Afterschool Program in San Anselmo, California:

We provide nutritious snacks that are low in fat and sugar; such as fresh fruit and vegetables and water rather than fruit juices.

We encourage the children to bring lunches that emphasize fresh fruits, vegetables, whole grain breads and lowfat milk, meats, poultry, fish, and cheeses.

We discourage high-sugar foods such as candy, fruit rolls, cookies, cakes, fruit drinks and high-fat foods such as potato chips.

If you wish to bring a refreshment for your child's birthday, please make arrangements with the group teacher. Simple birthday finger foods are preferred.

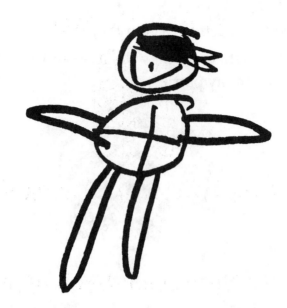

Ten Ways Parents Can Be Involved in Child Care or School Nutrition Programs

Everyone benefits when parents are able to contribute some of their time and ideas to the nutrition component in a child care or school setting. What can they do? Well, here are a few ideas:

- ❏ Help to establish or update statements of philosophy or policies
- ❏ Participate in planning the menus (within established guidelines)
- ❏ Take turns cooking lunch
- ❏ Contribute recipes for foods their children particularly like
- ❏ Act as chaperones for nutrition-related field trips
- ❏ Work with groups of children on cooking projects
- ❏ Make materials for nutrition learning activities
- ❏ Collect appropriate food packages and other props to be used in role-playing activities
- ❏ Be the supervising adults at meal tables
- ❏ Confer with caregivers or teachers about feeding problems

CHAPTER TWO

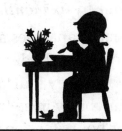

Feeding and Growth

Growth and the Nutritional Needs of Infants

❏ An infant will generally gain one ounce per day (about two pounds per month) during her first five months, and a half ounce per day (one pound per month) during the remainder of her first year.[1]

❏ By four to five months, a baby will generally double his birth weight, and by one year, he will triple it.[1]

❏ The average baby grows in length by 50% during the first year (that means that an infant who was 20 inches long at birth will be 30 inches long at one year).[1]

❏ Largely because of this rapid growth, infants have a greater need for calories, for each pound of body weight, than adults do.[1]

❏ Good nutrition is extremely important during this time, not just for general bodily growth, but for the infant's brain as well. The growth of the brain begins prior to birth, continues at a rapid pace into the child's second year, and is essentially complete by age six. In some cases, the brain can recover from the effects of poor nutrition if a good diet and stimulating environment are provided later, but not always.[2]

❏ In the first months of life, a baby can only swallow liquids, and has an immature digestive system that cannot handle the same foods older children can. *Breast milk or iron-fortified formula provides for essentially all of an infant's nutritional needs during the first four to six months of life.*[1]

❑ Infants have small stomach capacities and must eat more frequently than adults or older children. They should be fed "on demand," that is, when they indicate that they're hungry. You can expect some variability in eating patterns; a baby may be able to wait four hours for one feeding and then be hungry again two hours later.[1]

❑ Babies usually go through what doctors call "hungry periods." A common time for one of these periods is between 14 and 28 days of age.[1] Follow the baby's lead . . . if he's hungry more often than usual, feed him! He's probably getting ready for a growth spurt.

❑ Breast milk or formula generally provides enough water for a healthy young infant. If, however, a baby has diarrhea, or has been vomiting a lot, or the weather is very hot, she could become dehydrated if you don't offer her extra water. Once an infant starts eating solid foods, especially protein-rich foods like meats or egg yolks, she will need extra water to help her kidneys eliminate the waste products.[3] Keep in mind that babies sometimes cry because of thirst, not just hunger. *But never try to give an infant extra water by diluting her formula. And don't give a bottle of water as a pacifier; too much water can be as dangerous as too little.*

❑ Iron deficiency is one of the biggest nutritional problems among young children (read all about it in the section on *anemia* later in this book). The most critical time for making sure that a child has adequate iron intake is during the first year. The child will be building up a large blood supply in pace with her rapid growth. Children who do not consume adequate iron at this time are at greater risk for iron deficiency anemia during the toddler and preschool years.[4]

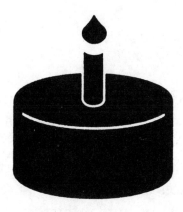

Different Ages, Different Stages . . . Infants

Stages of Infant Development[5] . . .	And Related Nutritional Considerations
1. She is attached to her primary caregivers.	1. She needs stable care, and she may refuse to accept feeding from strangers.
2. She will be developing a sense of trust about the world.	2. She is dependent on caregivers for her nourishment. She should be fed when she's hungry and allowed to stop eating when she's full. Weaning (from breast or bottle) should be a gradual process.
3. She uses her mouth to explore her environment.	3. She needs to be protected from hazards associated with choking and from poisonous substances.
4. She will be starting to view herself as a separate person. She needs to feel a sense of control over her environment.	4. She should be allowed to set the pace in feeding. She may refuse food in an attempt to get some sort of response from her caregiver.

Milks for the First Year

Young babies are really only equipped to swallow, digest, and obtain proper nourishment from milk. Even after infants are adept at eating solid foods, milk continues to be an important source of nutrients.[3] Breastmilk is the ideal first food for infants, but not all mothers want to breastfeed or have favorable circumstances for doing so.

Throughout a large part of human history, animal milks have been used as substitutes for mothers' milk. Cow's milk has been used most frequently, but goats, sheep, donkeys, horses, camels, pigs, deer, reindeer, and even dogs have been known to provide the milk that has fed human babies![6] It has only been recently, however, that substitute milks, or formulas, have come close to duplicating the nutritive qualities of breastmilk. Thanks to the wonders of modern technology, there are now three major types of commercially-prepared formulas that meet the specific needs of infants:[1]

Modified Cow's Milk Formulas (e.g., Similac®, Enfamil®)

Most babies who aren't breastfed get these formulas. The milk proteins have been altered to be more digestible, and vegetable oils provide the fat calories. Lactose is added to bring the carbohydrate levels up to that of human milk. Vitamins, minerals, and some other nutrients are added as well. These formulas are made with or without iron; iron-fortified formula is recommended.

Soy Formulas (e.g., Prosobee®, Isomil®)

These formulas are sometimes used for infants with allergies to cow's milk or infants who are sensitive to lactose after a bout with diarrhea (the carbohydrate in these formulas comes from sucrose or corn syrup).

Hypoallergenic Formulas (e.g., Pregestimil®, Nutramigen®)

Since some babies can tolerate neither cow's milk or soy milk, another variety of formula is available. These casein hydrolysate ("predigested") formulas don't smell or taste very good, and they are expensive, but for some infants they are the only option.

Whole cow's milk is inappropriate as a food for young infants. It is too high in protein and soluble salts, too low in iron and vitamin C, and can cause small amounts of gastrointestinal bleeding.[1] Most health experts recommend that infants drink breast milk or iron-fortified formula for the entire first year. However, the American Academy of Pediatrics has stated that it is all right to give an infant whole cow's milk after the age of six months, as long as he's getting at least a third of his calories from cereals, fruits, vegetables, and other foods that contain enough iron and vitamin C.[7] How do you know when that's happening? Well, he will probably be eating some table foods and should be eating at least:

❑ Six tablespoons of iron-fortified baby cereal

❑ Eight tablespoons of fruits and/or vegetables that are good sources of vitamin C

❑ Four tablespoons of meat or meat alternatives high in iron [8] (meat should usually be introduced to infants sometime between 8 to 10 months)

Lowfat (2%) and skim milk should not be given to children under the age of two. They are proportionately too low in fat and too high in protein to provide adequate nourishment for babies. *Infants should also not be given non-dairy creamers or imitation milks.*

Some commercial "weaning formulas" have appeared on the market recently. They give the impression that they are somehow advantageous for older babies, but in reality, they aren't.[9] They aren't harmful, either, but don't feel pressured to buy them.

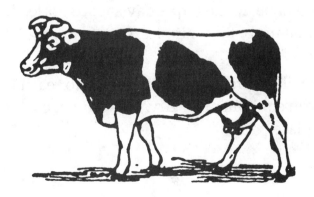

How to Prepare a Baby's Bottle

Select the Right Feeding

- ❏ You should only give a baby formula, breastmilk, milk (if he's old enough), and water from a bottle. Juices, cereals, and other solid foods or sweetened liquids do not belong in bottles.

- ❏ If you are using formula, get the iron-fortified variety. Babies need the iron, and contrary to popular belief, these formulas are no more likely to cause tummy upset than the varieties without iron.[4]

- ❏ If you will be using concentrated liquid or powdered formula, read the directions and measure carefully. It can be very dangerous for a baby to receive formula with too much or too little water in it.

- ❏ Check the expiration date on the container of formula, and reject cans that are bulging, badly dented, or rusty.

Make Sure Everything is Clean

- ❏ Wash your hands before preparing bottles.

- ❏ For babies up to three months of age, boil the water you will be using to mix the formula for five minutes.

- ❏ Use clean bottles:

  - • Wash the bottles, nipples, rings, and caps in hot, soapy water, using a brush to scrub all the nooks and crannies. Rinse in hot water.

  - • If you will be making up a day's worth of feedings at one time, boil the bottles, nipples, caps, and rings for five minutes.

  - • If you will be preparing bottles fresh for each feeding, let the clean equipment air-dry, then store it covered in a clean place.

- Wipe the top of the formula can with a clean, damp towel before you open it.
- Add formula for one feeding to each bottle, put the clean nipple in (upside down and with a cap on top if you'll be storing the bottle), and screw the ring on.
- Store prepared bottles for no more than 24 hours in the refrigerator; an open can of formula should be covered and used within 48 hours.

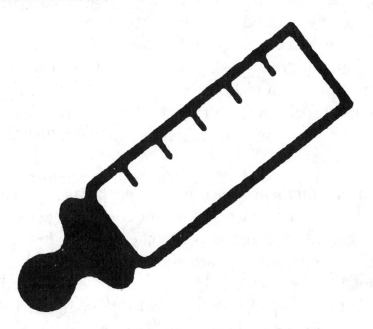

When It's Feeding Time

- Some babies will take a cold bottle; if you are going to warm the bottle, do it right before giving it to the baby.
- *Never heat a bottle in a microwave oven.* You can set the bottle in a bowl of warm water, hold it under warm running water from the faucet, or use a bottle-warming appliance.
- Before feeding the bottle to a baby, shake the formula or milk gently to mix it, and sprinkle a little onto your wrist to test its temperature.

How to Give a Bottle to a Baby

Feeding a bottle to a baby may seem like one of the simplest tasks around. Don't you just warm it up, stick the nipple in the baby's mouth, and stop when the milk is gone?

Well, actually, bottlefeeding doesn't always go so smoothly. Some babies are willing to go along with whatever happens; others may fuss, spit up a lot, or drink very little and be hungry again in a hour. When you are feeding a baby, remember that it is important, even at this early stage, for the child to feel relaxed and happy about eating. He will need to do this in order to be able to eat what he needs, as well as to begin a comfortable lifelong relationship with food. It is very easy to think of feeding as the process of making a baby drink a certain number of ounces of formula at a certain time. But what a baby really needs is to have his hunger satisfied when he feels it, and to experience the security of your love at the same time.

- ❏ *Feed an infant when she is hungry,* not because the clock says to. Some babies have characteristic cries or wiggles that let you know they're ready to eat; others may be fussier in general, and it may be harder to figure out what these babies want. It's worth checking to see if a baby has a wet diaper, needs to be burped, or just wants a little company. Once you've explored these possibilities, if she's still fussing, try feeding her.

- ❏ Gently get the baby settled down and comfortable for feeding.

- ❏ *Always hold a baby when giving a bottle.*
  - Hold his head higher than the rest of his body, so the milk doesn't flow into his inner ear and cause an infection.
  - Tip the bottle so milk fills the nipple and air doesn't get in.

- ❏ Wait for the baby to stop eating before you try to burp her. Then pat or rub her back gently while she rests on your shoulder or sits, supported with your other hand, on your lap.

❑ Avoid too many disruptions while you're feeding. Babies can get distracted or upset by a lot of burping, wiping, bouncing around, jiggling, and changing of positions.

❑ Pay attention to messages from the baby that he's full. He may:[1]

- close his lips
- stop sucking
- spit out the nipple
- turn his head away
- cover his mouth with his hands
- cry
- bite the nipple

Sometimes a baby will pause a bit (we all do, don't we?). Maybe he just needs a breather. Offer him the nipple again, but if he refuses it, he's probably had enough.

❑ Resist the temptation to make a baby finish the little bit of formula left in a bottle. Assume she knows her needs better than you do, and discard what's left. Rinse out the bottle with cool water to make cleaning easier later on.

How Child Care Providers Can Support Breastfeeding Moms

Because breastfeeding offers an infant so many advantages . . . just the right balance of nutrients, immune factors, and a special relationship . . . it is the recommended method of feeding infants today.[1] Many mothers face a challenge: they must return to work but would still like to be able to nurse their babies. There are several ways to manage breastfeeding and child care; an infant can be given breastmilk in a bottle, or the mother can nurse the baby in the child care setting during breaks from work, or the baby can be fed formula while in child care and breastfed at home.

If the mother will be nursing at the child care setting:

❑ Don't feed the baby for 1–1 1/2 hours before her mother is due to arrive, so that she will be hungry enough to nurse and keep up her mother's milk supply.

❑ Offer the mother a comfortable chair in a cozy place for nursing.[8]

If you will be feeding the baby breastmilk from a bottle, keep the milk safe:

❑ You can store breastmilk in the refrigerator for 48 hours or in the freezer for no more than two weeks after it has been expressed.

❑ Expressed milk should be stored in sterilized bottles or disposable plastic nursing bags.

❑ Do not allow the milk to sit at room temperature; take it from the refrigerator or freezer right before you will use it.

❑ Thaw the milk, if frozen, by running under cool, then very warm, water. Shake gently to mix (breastmilk separates during storage). *Do not warm breastmilk in a microwave oven!*

❑ Once breastmilk has thawed, do not refreeze.

❑ Discard unused portions.[8]

When Should a Baby Start Eating Solid Foods?

Breast milk or iron-fortified formula (perhaps with vitamin or mineral supplementation prescribed by a doctor) gives an infant all of the nutrients he needs for the first four to six months of life.

Some parents and caregivers want babies to eat solid foods as soon as possible. They may believe (mistakenly) that solid foods help young babies sleep through the night,[10] or they may want to prove that their children are truly "advanced." Other parents or caregivers may wait too long to introduce foods with new textures to babies. A time will come when a baby needs the nutritients and the challenges that solids provide; meanwhile there are good reasons to wait until the infant is developmentally ready to accept them:[8]

- ❑ Babies can choke on foods they can't swallow easily.
- ❑ Some foods are difficult for young infants to digest.
- ❑ Babies can develop food allergies when they're exposed to certain foods too early.
- ❑ When babies start eating solid foods, they cut back on breast milk or formula, which is their *ideal* source of nutrients for the first four to six months.

Suppose a baby is five months old and you're wondering if it's time for her to try some infant cereal. How will you know she's ready? In general she should be able to:[8]

- ❑ hold her neck steady and sit with support
- ❑ draw in her lower lip when a spoon is removed from her mouth
- ❑ keep food in her mouth and swallow it
- ❑ open her mouth when she sees food coming

It is very important that parents and child care providers communicate with each other and agree on their approach to this transitional time. You will need to discuss *what* is to be introduced as well as when to start. Many parents want to be the first to experience these developmental changes with their babies.

A Solid-Food Itinerary for Baby

The solid foods you offer a baby should give her two things: needed nutrients and opportunities to develop her eating skills. Hopefully by the end of her first year, she will be feeding herself soft table food and drinking from a cup. During the transition from exclusive nipple-feeding to a more adult eating pattern, she will become accustomed to a wide range of flavors and textures in a relatively short time. It's really quite an accomplishment!

We agree with child-feeding expert Ellyn Satter, who asserts that the best way to get through this time is to start solids late and move quickly into table foods.[10] We recommend that you read *Child of Mine: Feeding With Love and Good Sense* for the finer details of feeding infants. Meanwhile, we've adapted information from her book to give you general guidelines regarding solid foods for babies.

> **Age:** 4–7 months
> **Nutritional needs:** Iron
> **Feeding skills:** Swallowing smooth semi-solid foods
> **New food:** Iron-fortified infant cereal

Start with infant rice cereal, which is the least likely to cause allergies, and mix it with formula, breastmilk, or diluted evaporated milk. Wait a week, then try barley, then oats. It is recommended that you wait until a baby is eight or nine months old before you give him wheat cereals, because wheat commonly causes allergies.

We don't recommend that you give a young infant regular oatmeal or other adult hot cereals, simply because they don't have enough available iron. And don't buy jars of fruit mixed with infant cereal; it's hard to tell how much cereal is in them. Please, never add sugar or other sweeteners to baby's cereal. He doesn't know cereal is supposed to taste sweet, and what he doesn't know will be good for him!

Experiment to find the right consistency for the cereal mixture; some babies like it thin and some like it thick. Eventually the baby should be eating about a half-cup of cereal mixture, divided between two meals. It is recommended that children continue eating these iron-fortified infant cereals for at least the first year and perhaps up to the age of eighteen months.[11]

At this point, you should not be trying to replace milk feedings; rather cereal should be a supplement to them.

```
Age: 6–8 months
Nutritional needs: Vitamin A, vitamin C
Feeding skills: Moving tongue from side to
                side, controlling swallow,
                beginning up and down
                munching motion, curving lips
                around a cup
New foods:      Fruits and vegetables, pureed or
                mashed, later, juice in a cup
```

It doesn't really matter whether you introduce fruits or vegetables first. Very ripe, mashed bananas are often recommended as a first fruit for babies, but they aren't good sources of either vitamin A or C. Be sure to try sweet potatoes, squash, peaches, apricots, spinach, carrots, purple plums, broccoli, cauliflower, cantaloupe, strawberries, and potatoes.

You can puree cooked vegetables or tender fruits in a baby-food grinder or you can mash the foods with a fork, depending on the food and the eating skills of the child. Avoid canned vegetables, which are usually high in sodium, and canned or frozen fruits with added sugar. Commercial baby fruits are fortified with vitamin C and may be a convenient option for you. The only problem with them is that they are so smooth and thin that they don't challenge a baby to learn about new textures.

Wait at least three days to check for an allergic reaction before introducing the next food. Common reactions are hives, rashes, vomiting, diarrhea, coughing, or excessive gas.

At this time it's wise to limit fruits and vegetables to four tablespoons per day. This is to make sure the baby doesn't fill up on these foods and refuse those with greater nutrient density. It's also a good idea to limit high-nitrate foods like carrots (especially carrot juice), beets, collards, and spinach to a tablespoon or two per serving until the baby is older.

Breastmilk or formula should still be providing most of a baby's nutrition at this age. But she is building up experience with tastes and textures, which is important for the next step.

Age: 7–10 months
Nutritional needs: Protein, vitamins, minerals
Feeding skills: Chewing, grasping food in palm of hand and later, fingers, drinking from a cup
New foods: Modified table foods . . . lumpy fruits and vegetables, finger breads and cereals, milk in a cup, ground meats, flaked fish, cottage cheese, grated cheese, and yogurt, cooked dried beans (mashed), tofu, pasta

---

When an infant has mastered mashed fruits and vegetables, you can let him try to feed himself dry cereals like Cheerios as a snack, or let him gnaw at a breadstick. This is a good time to introduce him to milk in a cup.

Some experts suggest that you wait until a baby is a year old before you give him citrus fruits. If he isn't predisposed to allergies, though, it's probably okay to give him an orange or grapefruit wedge now and see what happens. Many babies enjoy these tart fruits, and they are excellent sources of vitamin C.

By the time a baby is eight months old, he will be able to eat many table foods, and the real fun begins! Meats are introduced at this point and should be finely ground at first. It helps to moisten the meat with gravy, milk, or some other liquid. Meat is also popular mixed into mashed potatoes or in casseroles with pasta. Later on you can chop the meat finely.

Plain commercial baby meats are another option, if you happen to be making something for everyone else that would be obviously inappropriate for a baby. Work up to about an ounce of meat or the equivalent of a meat alternative every day.

> **Meat Equivalents**[12]
>
> 1 oz. beef, lamb, poultry
> 1 oz. cheese (1/4 c. grated)
> 1/2 c. cooked dried beans
> 1/4 c. cottage cheese
> 1/4 c. flaked tuna or salmon
> 4 oz. tofu (does not meet Child Care
>   Food Program Guidelines)

Babies can easily choke when they try to eat foods that are too advanced in texture for them. Be especially careful not to give babies foods that can form hard plugs in their throats, like raw hard vegetable or fruit chunks, nuts, tough meats, hot dogs, and anything with bones or pits. Hard candies and snack chips are dangerous, and have no place in their diet anyway.

> **These foods should be avoided for**
> **children less than a year old**[8]
>
> salt, sugar, heavy seasonings
> chocolate (*allergies*)
> egg whites (*allergies*)
> shellfish (*allergies*)
> peanut butter (*choking*)
> honey, even in cooked goods
>   (*infant botulism*)

How to Feed Solid Foods to a Baby

We said earlier that *how* you feed is as important as *what* you feed. Both you and baby will have an easier go of it if you keep the following guidelines in mind when feeding solid foods.[8,10] Call on all your reserves of patience and humor, and realize that even when baby ends up with more squash in his hair than in his mouth, he will think it's a terrific experience if you do!

❑ Feed a baby only when he's sitting up; if he can't sit up yet, he's not ready for solid foods.

❑ When you first offer solids (usually cereals), try them only at one meal a day to get the baby used to the idea of spoon feeding. Serve only a teaspoon or two of a new food at first. You can add more meals and bigger servings later.

❑ In the beginning, feed the baby a little breastmilk or formula first, so he'll be patient but not stuffed. By the time he is eight or ten months old and eating table foods, you can skip the milk feeding before the meal entirely.

❑ Wash your hands and the baby's hands before feeding time.

❑ Try to keep the atmosphere as tranquil as possible. Sit facing the baby and be friendly but not too entertaining.

❑ Test the food first to make sure it isn't too hot.

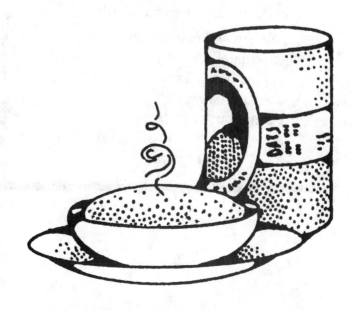

❏ Offer the food on a small spoon and wait for baby's mouth to open. Place a small amount of food between the baby's lips; he may force it out of his mouth, in which case it's okay to scoop it up and try again. However, if he doesn't seem to like it, respect his preference.

❏ Some babies need a lot of exposure to certain foods before they like them. If a baby refuses a food, try it again some other time.

❏ Stop feeding the baby when he lets you know he's full. He may:[1]

- close his mouth
- turn his head away
- spit out food
- cover his mouth with his hands
- play with utensils
- cry
- shake his head "no"
- hand you the bowl or cup

❏ When a baby grabs the spoon from you and tries to feed himself, or when he wants to eat (or explore) the food with his fingers, stay out of the way and enjoy the show!

❏ Keep the food safe:

- Don't feed right out of a baby food jar (unless you're willing to throw out the leftovers).
- Throw out what baby hasn't eaten if his spoon has touched the food.
- Store opened jars of baby food in the refrigerator for no longer than three days.

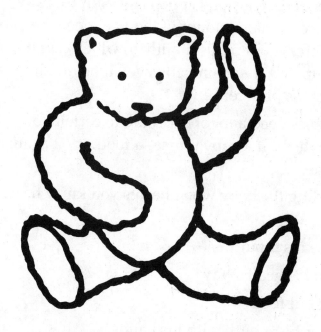

How to Prevent Baby Bottle Tooth Decay

We have met young children whose teeth were so rotten that it was painful for them to eat. They were suffering from "baby bottle tooth decay." Cavities formed in their primary ("baby") teeth when these children were put to bed with bottles containing milk, formula, juice, or other sweetened liquids. Such children endure unnecessary discomfort and may require expensive dental work.

Baby bottle tooth decay can be prevented by:[8]

- ❏ using bottles to feed infants breastmilk, formula, milk, or water *only.*

- ❏ offering bottles only at feeding times, not before naps or bedtime. If the baby falls asleep anyway, move him around a bit to stimulate swallowing; this will move at least some of the milk out of the mouth.

- ❏ not dipping pacifiers in honey, maple syrup, or corn syrup.

- ❏ putting a baby to bed with stuffed animals, lullabyes, or back rubs, not bottles.

- ❏ serving juice to a baby in a cup, not a bottle.

Weaning a Baby from Breast or Bottle

Weaning is ideally a *gradual* transition from milk feeding by nipple to a varied diet with milk drunk from a cup. We aren't going to argue here that one time is better than another for the completion of this process. Some parents are in no particular hurry to see their children off the breast or bottle, some children refuse to give up nipple feeding (and their parents have to endure remarks like "is he planning to go off to college with that bottle?"), and some children lose interest in breast- or bottlefeeding as soon as they figure out how to drink from a cup.

We believe every family has to find their own best solution to this dilemma. If you are interested in pursuing the topic further, we suggest you read about it in *Child of Mine: Feeding with Love and Good Sense*.[10]

What is important is that a child be well-established on table foods by the age of ten or twelve months. She won't receive adequate nutrition if milk remains the major component of her diet past this point. After the age of one (and until the preteen years), two cups of milk a day is sufficient; she should be getting the rest of her calories from a variety of other foods selected from the "four food groups."

Get the baby used to drinking liquids from a cup by offering small amounts of juice, formula, milk, or water by cup when she's around seven or eight months old. She'll need your help at the time, of course, but with the right equipment (plastic cups with two handles are dandy) and lots of practice, in a couple of months she'll be able to manage drinking milk at mealtime by herself. By then, if breastfeeding or a bottle is offered, it should be only at snacks, or in the early morning or late evening. Eventually, as the child is eating more and more like the rest of the family or group, these milk feedings can be dropped, one at a time. Usually the child will scarcely notice what's happened.

Remember, do not let a child of any age go to sleep with a bottle.

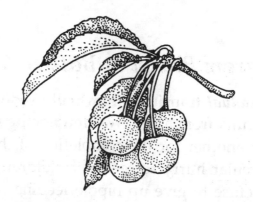

Growth and the Nutritional Needs of Toddlers

❑ Toddlers don't grow as rapidly as infants. For the next several years, they will be gaining about three inches and four to six pounds a year.[1]

❑ By the end of the second year, a child's brain has reached 75% of its adult size.[1]

❑ By the age of 2 1/2 years, a child usually has all twenty "baby teeth."[2] Even though these teeth don't have to last a lifetime, they are important for proper chewing. Young children need to learn how to care for their teeth, and they should be offered foods that don't promote cavities. Also, the nutrients taken in during the childhood years will affect the health of the permanent teeth.[13]

❑ Iron deficiency and its late stage, anemia, can be problems among toddlers. Especially at risk are children who didn't get enough iron while they were infants, and those who drink too much milk and eat too few iron-rich foods.[4]

❑ It is *normal* for toddlers to have erratic appetites or to go on "food jags." An example of a food jag is when a child wants nothing but macaroni and cheese for two weeks, then abruptly wants nothing to do with the stuff. Does this sound like anyone you know? Despite these problems, most toddlers manage to grow pretty well.[2]

❑ Some children at this age are fond of eating non-food items like dirt, paint chips, paper, and crayons. Dirt and paint chips can cause lead poisoning, so discourage them from eating these at least.[2]

Different Ages, Different Stages . . . Toddlers

How a Toddler is Developing . . .[5]

1. He has an expanding sense of self, as a separate person.

2. He is becoming able to express himself verbally.

3. He is involved in intensive exploration of the world around him and needs both the freedom to explore and the security of limits.

4. He is refining his fine motor control, but may be easily frustrated by setbacks.

5. He is neophobic (afraid of anything new) . . . Nature probably installed this tendency in toddlers to protect them!

6. He has a short attention span.

And Related Nutritional Considerations

1. He loves to say "NO" and may refuse to eat even favorite foods as a way of establishing control.

2. He can tell you when he's hungry and what he likes to eat.

3. He may be more interested in playing than in eating.
   He will play with his food as a way of learning about it.
   He needs limits in the form of established meals and snack times and expectations regarding behavior at the table.

4. He needs to be set up for success in self-feeding, with the right utensils and seating, and food that's easy to handle. If you are too fussy about tidiness at this point, you could delay the development of his feeding skills.

5. He will almost certainly refuse to try a new food, at least once!

6. He may not be able to sit through a long meal.

How to Survive Mealtime With Young Children (and Perhaps Even Enjoy It)

- ❑ Allow enough time for an unhurried meal.

- ❑ Let the children know in advance what kind of behavior you expect.

- ❑ Set aside a little quiet time before the meal, maybe reading a story or having them listen to some music.

- ❑ See that the children are comfortably seated and have the right equipment for eating.

- ❑ Respect the children's preferences when planning meals, but don't give in to "short-order cooking."

- ❑ Offer new foods in a matter-of-fact way along with some familiar foods, like bread.

- ❑ Allow the children to participate in food preparation.

- ❑ Don't allow them to fill up on juice or milk throughout the day.

- ❑ Help the children to *serve themselves* small portions, and be ready to help them with seconds later.

- ❑ Present food in a form that's easy for children to manage (see *Modifying Foods for Children of Different Ages*, page 59).

- ❑ Acknowledge desirable behavior and ignore undesirable behavior. Don't, however, praise or reward a child for eating or for trying new foods. Act as though you assume she is able to handle the situation, and she will (eventually).

- ❑ Do not make desserts the reward for eating the rest of the meal. Make them *nutritious* and offer them with the other foods. If they're eaten first, so what?

- ❑ Set a good example by eating a wide variety of foods and being open to trying new ones.

Young Children Eat Better When They Have the Right Equipment (for feeding)

Picture yourself sitting in a chair that leaves your feet dangling three feet from the ground, at a table that reaches to your neck, trying to spear pieces of cauliflower with a fork that's two feet long. Would eating be enjoyable?

Well, eating with adult-size utensils at adult-size furniture feels like this to a young child. If children are going to be comfortable enough to sit through meals and successful enough at feeding themselves to feel good about it, they will need utensils they can handle and a thoughtfully set up environment. A bonus for you will be less mess to contend with.

❏ Chairs should have supports for children's feet or allow the children to have their feet on the floor.

❏ The table should be at a height that allows children to easily reach their food and eat it.

❏ Plates, bowls, glasses, cups, and flatware should be child-sized and made of unbreakable materials.

❏ Plates with curved sides are easier for younger children to work with. Glasses should have broad bases and be small enough to allow children to get their hands around them.

❏ Spoons should have short handles, blunt tips, and rounded bowls. Forks should have short handles and short, blunt tines. Knives should be small and have rounded tips. Disposable flatware isn't recommended except for picnics.

❏ Children can enjoy pouring their own beverages if you provide small (covered) pitchers with broad handles.

❏ When you're serving family-style meals, keep the serving spoons small enough for children to manage, too.

❏ Children with handicapping conditions may require specialized eating equipment.

Growth and the Nutritional Needs of Preschoolers

❑ Preschoolers are growing pretty much at the same rate they did as toddlers . . . approximately three inches and four to six pounds a year.[13]

❑ The nutritional concerns for preschoolers are much the same as for toddlers, too. Iron deficiency anemia is still a problem, although it gets less common as children get older. Tooth decay and obesity are significant health problems in this age group.[15]

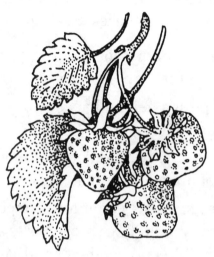

❑ Young preschoolers still display some of the eating behaviors that so worried their parents when they were toddlers: finickiness, erratic appetites, and dawdling at the table. By the time they're four or five, though, most of these children will be eating pretty well and be good company at mealtimes.[2]

Different Ages, Different Stages . . . Preschoolers

How a Preschooler is Developing . . .[5]

And Related Nutritional Considerations

1. Her ability to master skills more easily makes her eager to cooperate and try new experiences. She does need immediate reinforcement of her success to stay interested, however.

1. She will probably be more willing to try new foods.

    You can still expect some messiness while she eats, but she will be trying hard to imitate grown-up eating. She still needs to be set up for success, with the proper equipment and thoughtful food preparation.

2. She is becoming less attached to her primary caregiver, and expands her relationships with peers, family members, and other adults.

2. She will be influenced by the food preferences of her peers and teachers or caregivers.

3. She is learning to feel positively or negatively about herself, depending upon her interactions with others.

3. Her own food preferences should be respected.

    She needs to know that people care enough about her to attend to her basic needs (like food).

    She feels important when she helps out and will enjoy preparing food for herself and others.

The Most Important Things You Can Do to Help Children Grow Up Having Their Own "Best Bodies"

Foster a Positive Self-Image

❑ Provide an environment in which children can learn to appreciate the richness of diversity . . . in body sizes, skin colors, cultural backgrounds, abilities, and the like.

❑ Remember that children need limits, opportunities to develop self-reliance, and lots of love.

❑ Be alert to the need for counseling when things aren't going well in the family.

Encourage Lots of Physical Activity

❑ Set limits on television watching.

❑ Don't carry a child who can walk.

❑ Provide a safe play environment outside, with opportunities to use a variety of muscles . . . pulling, pushing, climbing, jumping, and running.

❑ Walk with children instead of driving, when you can.

❑ When it's stormy weather, dance or put on a kids' exercise video.

❑ Don't just sit there . . . play along!

Promote Healthful Eating Habits

❑ Make a variety of foods available, generally avoiding those with excessive sugar and fat, and establish *regular* meal and snack times.

❑ Allow children to decide whether and how much to eat.

❑ Don't single out the overweight child with special foods or restrictions.

❑ Encourage children to eat slowly and appreciatively.

❑ Never use food as a reward or withhold food as punishment.

❑ Be a good role model by eating healthfully and staying out of the "dieting" trap.

George Won't Eat His Broccoli?
Melissa Won't Even Look at a Snow Pea?
Here, Try This . . .

❑ Let him grow it.

❑ Let her help you pick it out at the grocery store or farmers' market.

❑ Let him help you prepare it for eating (even quite young children can shell peas, pop beans, separate broccoli florets, and wash lettuce).

❑ Try serving it a different way . . . raw if you usually cook it, lightly steamed if you usually serve it raw, perhaps even pureed in a soup.

❑ Let him dip it (see recipes for some healthful dips, pages 110–11)

❑ Put parmesan cheese on top.

❑ Give it a funny name.

❑ Serve it when she's hungry, not when she's filled up on other stuff.

❑ Seat him next to a child who *loves* vegetables and let peer pressure work its magic.

❑ Tell her she can have it for dessert, but only if she eats all of her cupcake (just kidding . . .).

❑ Eat it yourself, with obvious enjoyment.

❑ Don't assume he'll *never* like it. Some children take longer than others to feel comfortable with certain foods, so let it reappear occasionally.

❑ If a young child still won't eat vegetables, and you are concerned that her health will suffer, offer her fruits that are good sources of vitamins A and C (see lists, pages 70–71).

Calvin and Hobbes
by Bill Watterson

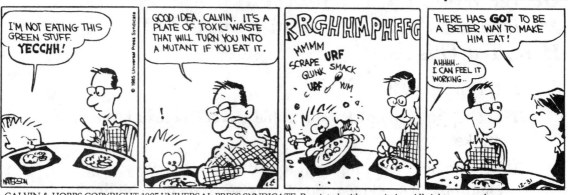

Growth and the Nutritional Needs of School-Age Children

❏ Up to about seven or eight years of age, children will be gaining their usual three inches per year in height and four to six pounds in weight. Then they'll slow down a bit, gaining about two inches a year, until they start their adolescent growth spurts (the spurt can happen as early as nine in girls).[13]

❏ Between six years and puberty, boys are taller and heavier than girls. By the sixth grade, it's not unusual to find classrooms in which most of the girls are bigger than most of the boys (by sometime in high school, the boys regain their size advantage).[13]

❏ It is *normal* for children to put on some weight before they experience their spurt in height. Tragically, many children, or their parents, become so concerned about this that dieting and weight obsession start at this young age.[16]

❏ Feeding problems are uncommon among six- to twelve-year olds, as children gradually become more accepting of what is served to them.[15] However, as parents lose some of the control over what their children are eating, many children make poor food choices. One study found that school-age children were getting 25% of their calories from *sugar*![17]

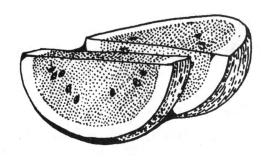

Different Ages, Different Stages . . . School-Age Children

How the School-age Child is Developing[15] . . .	And Related Nutritional Considerations
1. He experiences mastery of physical skills and may become involved in organized sports.	**1.** He will probably have a hearty appetite.
2. He is increasingly influenced by peers and the school enviroment.	**2.** He may start to question his parents' (or caregiver's) crediblity. Nutrition education activities may be part of the classroom curriculum.
3. He has more access to money and opportunities for shopping without parents.	**3.** He can buy foods on his own, some of which may not be acceptable to parents and caregivers.
4. He may have a hectic schedule as he becomes more involved in activities outside the home.	**4.** He may skip meals, especially breakfast.
5. He may spend large amounts of time watching television.	**5.** Watching television can contribute to obesity;[18] advertising may encourage children to eat unhealthful foods.

Helping Older Children Make Better Eating Choices

Children become increasingly independent as they progress from kinder-garten to junior high. They enjoy learning to make decisions for them-selves, and eating behavior is one area over which they can exert some control. As money and opportunities become available, school-age children obtain access to foods their parents and schools or child care settings don't provide. And often the foods they choose to eat are, well, not exactly what you'd call nutritious!

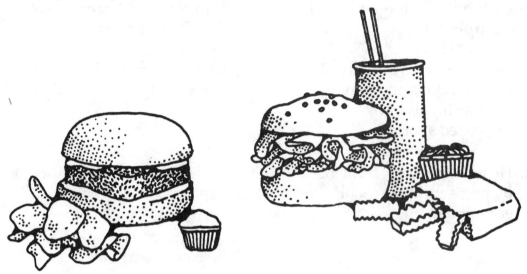

These "junk" foods aren't going to go away, and so long as they're around, kids will want to eat them. So how can you support a child in thinking for himself, yet keep him from turning into a veritable candy-eating machine?

❑ Remember that it is still your job to determine what will be served to a child while he is in your home or child care setting, and at what time. It is still the child's job to decide whether to eat or how much to eat.[16] You may not be able to control what a child eats when he's not with you, but at least you can be assured he's getting nutritious food when he is with you. And hopefully, he will enjoy a wide range of healthful foods.

❑ Include the children in your menu-planning process. Let them know what the guidelines have to be (servings from particular food groups, restrictions on sugar, fat, or salt, or whatever). Explain to them the reasons for the guidelines. Then try to accommodate as many of their suggestions as possible. They will feel very important, and they'll be getting nutrition education at the same time.

❑ Involve the children in food preparation. As children get older they usually end up fixing more of their own meals and snacks. Teach them some simple but nutritious recipes (you can make your own laminated recipe cards with pictures); eventually you'll be able to set out the ingredients and let them do all the work! By the way, it's as important for boys to learn to cook as it is for girls.

❑ Teach children to be informed consumers. Discuss how television advertising, prizes, and packaging can lead people to make unwise food choices. Have them read food labels. Make games of finding cereals with the least sugar, or the lowest-fat crackers.

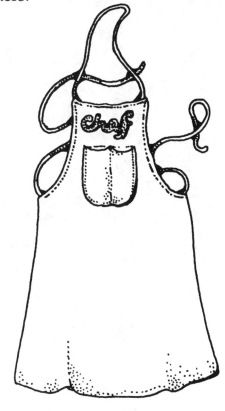

PART TWO

Your Feeding Program

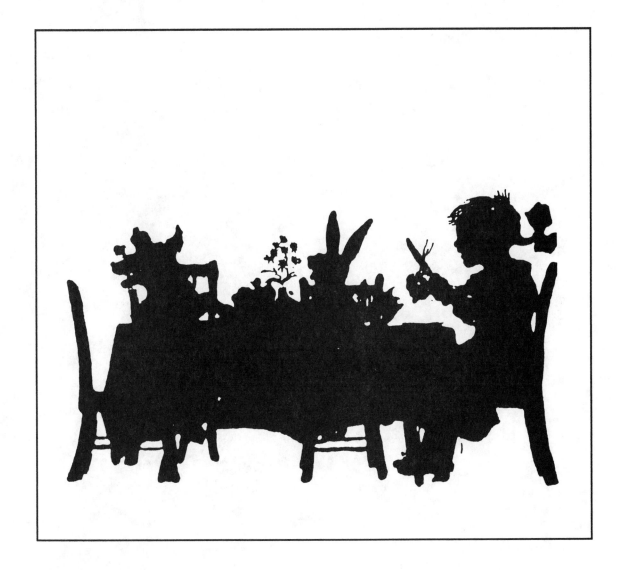

CHAPTER THREE

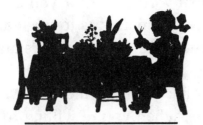

Planning How and What to Feed Children

Why Bother With a Feeding Program?

We feel that it's beneficial to everyone if a child's meals while in child care are provided by the caregiver. There are many reasons for this:

❑ Some of the mealtime disturbances that occur when a few children bring "junk" foods, or when food items are traded, can be avoided.

❑ Children will, in general, get more variety and nutrient balance in their meals . . . bag lunches tend to be pretty much the same day after day, in part because they are limited to foods that travel well.

❑ You can make mealtimes valuable learning experiences, when you introduce children to foods they might otherwise never encounter, or can talk about foods that everyone is eating.

❑ Parents are usually extremely grateful to be spared the hassle of packing lunches.

Despite the advantages, however, you must realistically look at your situation, that is, the space, equipment, and time you have available, before you decide whether to offer a full meal program or snacks only. We don't want you to make yourself and everyone else miserable because you've taken on more than you can handle!

You may find that what works best for you is to offer snacks only, but in combination with a specific policy as to what are acceptable bag lunch foods. (For example, some child care providers and schools have policies that forbid sodas, candy, or other sugary foods in lunches brought from home). It is certainly possible to offer children a wide range of food experiences during snack times, when you're willing to move beyond crackers and juice (we'll show you how later on). Parents may appreciate having a copy of *Your Faithful Lunchbox Guide* (page 73) to help them plan bag lunches.

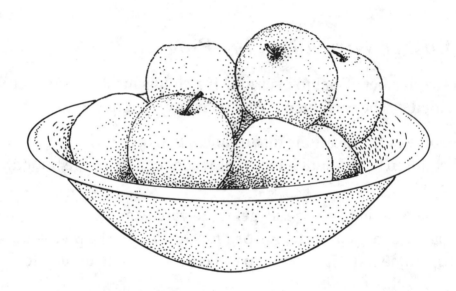

We also suggest that you look into signing up for the Child Care Food Program (CCFP)*, if you haven't already. Qualified providers can get CCFP reimbursement for meals and snacks served in child care homes and centers, plus good training opportunities and support. We have followed the meal patterns and serving size requirements of the program while developing the recipes for this book, to make it easier for you to meet their guidelines.

*Check the white pages in your phone directory for "Child Care Food Program."

How to Serve Meals

There are several ways to set up a meal for children, and you may find that it's fun to vary your usual routine now and then. We don't recommend serving children meals already portioned out on plates if you can possibly help it, because it doesn't allow them to decide for themselves how much they want to eat. You may also find that a lot of food is wasted this way. There are better ways to serve meals, and we've outlined them below.

Family Style

Meal tables are set up with plates, flatware, and cups at each place, and the food is passed in small bowls, plates, or baskets from which the children help themselves. Beverages are served in small pitchers so the children can pour for themselves.

This is the recommended method for serving most meals to children and can be used even with toddlers; very young children may need more assistance getting the food on their plates, however.

Buffet Style

Foods are placed in serving dishes on one table or counter, and children move along serving themselves from what's offered. This serving method is not recommended for very young children, but you may find it works well with older kids just as a change of pace, for snacks, or for special occasions.

Be particularly careful that the children are capable of handling the food and utensils in a hygenic manner.

Picnics

You can serve these meals outside at picnic tables or on blankets, or even inside on a blanket if it's a cold or rainy day. Pack up the food items in a basket or insulated chest, being especially careful to keep foods at safe temperatures should you be traveling farther than your back yard.

Whatever style you choose, remember that an adult should always eat with the children.

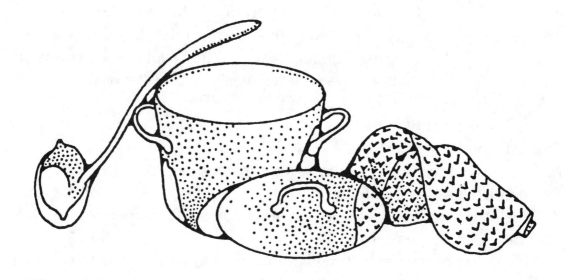

Reminders for Adults at Mealtime

❑ Adults should eat meals and snacks with the children (the **same** meals and snacks, unless you have a medical or religious reason for avoiding certain foods, which should then be explained to the children).

❑ Make sure everyone has washed hands, is comfortably seated, and has all the proper utensils.

❑ Help the children serve themselves small portions from the serving bowls and be ready to assist children with second helpings.

❑ Keep the conversation at the table light; avoid nagging, criticism, and other unpleasantries, and don't allow fighting or rudeness.

❑ It's okay to talk about the foods being served (where they come from, what their sensory characteristics are, or why they might be healthful to eat).

❑ Respect children's food preferences; resist the temptation to interfere, using such tactics as rewarding children for trying new foods or forcing them to clean their plates.

❑ Expect everyone to sit down at the table to participate in the meal, but allow children who finish early to leave the table and engage in some quiet activity like reading (after they've done their part in cleanup, of course).

❑ Do *not* allow children to watch television while eating.

❑ Remember that you are a role model for good eating behaviors and enjoyment; be willing to try new foods, eat at least a little of all of the meal components, and remember to say please and thank you.

Your job is to[1]

• make the meal pleasant
• help the children participate in the meal
• allow eating methods appropriate for the developmental levels of the children
• enforce standards of behavior

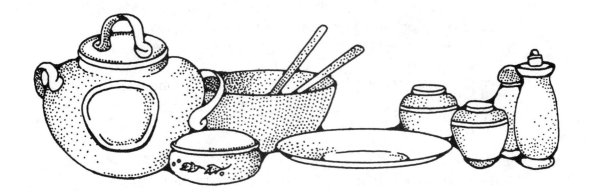

How to Plan Menus

A well-planned menu is a time- and money-saving tool for you, a powerful nutrition education message to children and parents, and makes it much more likely that the children will get the best nourishment you can provide. Busy families, too, find that planning menus ahead means fewer annoying trips to the store, better meals, and more time to enjoy each other! It seems intimidating at first, but we'll run you through it, step-by-step.

❑ Gather all of your tools together: menu form or pad of paper, pencil, cookbooks and recipes, a guide to seasonal fruits and vegetables, information on current prices of various food items, lists of foods high in vitamins A and C and iron, a calendar of holidays or special events, and the menu checklist. Menu forms (like the one we've included on page 122) make it easy to remember to plan servings of all the required food groups.

❑ Decide the time period of your menu. Some cooks like to plan for a month at a time and then start over; some find that repeating "cycles" of three to four weeks work best. Families and small child care settings may prefer weekly menu planning.

❑ Think about the staff, equipment, time, and storage space you have available.

❑ Figure out how you want to approach planning the meals. You may want to plan breakfasts, lunches, and snacks for one entire day before moving on to the next day. Many people find it helpful to plan all of the main dishes for the time period, then all of the grain items, and so on. It's usually a good idea to plan snacks last, so that you can use them to fill in the nutritional gaps left by the breakfasts and lunches.

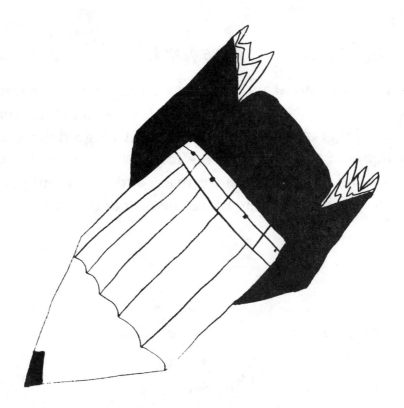

❑ As discussed earlier, you may need to plan adjustments in preparation methods, or even alternative items, in order to accommodate different age groups.

❑ Consider the time between snacks and meals when you plan snacks. If it will be three hours until the next meal, the snack should be more substantial (preferably with a protein-rich food included) than one which precedes a meal by an hour and a half. You want the children hungry at mealtime, but not frantically so.

❑ Use the menu checklist to see how you did.

❑ Check which ingredients you have on hand, then make up your shopping list or purchase orders.

Serving Size Guidelines for Child Care

The most convenient way to ensure that you're providing adequate amounts of nutrients to children is to plan meals that conform to the Child Care Food Program requirements.* **The CCFP guidelines call for a specified number of servings from the four major food groups: milk, meat or meat alternatives, breads and cereals, and fruits and vegetables.** We've printed them for your reference on the next two pages.

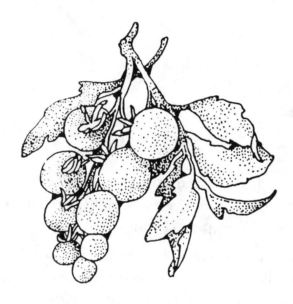

To do the best possible job of planning meals for children, you should become familiar with the Dietary Guidelines for Americans (page 61) and the good food sources of important nutrients (pages 70–72). You may also find it helpful to review *Appendix A—Nutrition Basics.*

*If you participate in the School Lunch Program, you will need to follow its guidelines, of course.

Infant and Child Meal Patterns

Food Components	Birth through 3 months	4–7 months	8–11 months
Breakfast	4–6 fluid ounces (fl. oz.) breast milk[1] or formula[2]	4–8 fl. oz. breast milk[1] or formula[2] 0–3 Tbl. infant cereal[3] (optional)	6–8 fl. oz. breast milk,[1] formula[2] or whole milk 2–4 Tbl. infant cereal[3] 1–4 Tbl. fruit *and/or* vegetable
Lunch or Supper	4–6 fl. oz. breast milk[1] or formula[2]	4–8 fl. oz. breast milk[1] or formula[2] 0–3 Tbl. infant cereal[3] (optional) 0–3 Tbl. fruit *and/or* vegetable (optional)	6–8 fl. oz. breast milk,[1] formula[2] or whole milk 2–4 Tbl. infant cereal[3] *and/or* 1–4 Tbl. meat, fish, poultry, egg yoke or cooked dry beans or peas, *or* 1/2–2 oz. cheese, *or* 1–4 oz. cottage cheese, cheese food or cheese spread 1–4 Tbl. fruit *and/or* vegetable
Snack	4–6 fl. oz. breast milk[1] or formula[2]	4–6 fl. oz. breast milk[1] or formula[2]	2–4 fl. oz. breast milk[1] formula,[2] whole milk or fruit juice[4] 0–1/2 slice bread *or* 0–2 crackers[5] (optional)

[1] Meals containing only breast milk are not reimbursable
[2] Iron-fortified infant formula
[3] Iron-fortified dry infant cereal
[4] Full strength fruit juice
[5] Made from whole grain or enriched meal or flour

Food Components	Ages 1 to 3 years	Ages 3 to 6 years	Ages 6–12 years
Breakfast			
1. Milk, fluid	1/2 cup	3/4 cup	1 cup
2. Vegetable, fruit or full-strength juice	1/4 cup	1/2 cup	1/2 cup
3. Bread and bread alternates (whole grain or enriched):			
Bread	1/2 slice	1/2 slice	1 slice
or cornbread, rolls, muffins, or biscuits	1/2 serving	1/2 serving	1 serving
or cold dry cereal (volume or weight, whichever is less)	1/4 cup or 1/3 oz.	1/3 cup or 1/2 oz.	3/4 cup or 1 oz.
or cooked cereal, pasta, noodle products, or cereal grains	1/4 cup	1/4 cup	1/2 cup
Lunch or Supper			
1. Milk, fluid	1/2 cup	3/4 cup	1 cup
2. Vegetable and/or fruit (2 or more kinds)	1/4 cup total	1/2 cup total	3/4 cup total
3. Bread and bread alternates (whole grain or enriched):			
Bread	1/2 slice	1/2 slice	1 slice
or cornbread, rolls, muffins, or biscuits	1/2 serving	1/2 serving	1 serving
or cooked cereal, pasta, noodle products, or cereal grains	1/4 cup	1/4 cup	1/2 cup
4. Meat or meat alternates	1 oz.	1-1/2 oz.	2 oz.
Lean meat, fish, or poultry (edible portion as served)			
or cheese or cottage cheese	1 oz.	1-1/2 oz.	2 oz.
or egg	1 egg	1 egg	1 egg
or cooked dry beans or peas[1]	1/4 cup	3/8 cup	1/2 cup
or peanut butter, soy nut butter, or other nut or seed butters	2 Tbsps.	3 Tbsps.	4 Tbsps.
or peanuts, soy nuts, tree nuts, or seeds[2]	1/2 oz.[3]	3/4 oz.[3]	1 oz.[3]
or an equivalent quantity of any combination of the above meat/meat alternates			
AM or PM Supplement (Select 2 of these 4 components.)[4]			
1. Milk, fluid	1/2 cup	1/2 cup	1 cup
2. Vegetable, fruit, or full-strength juice	1/2 cup	1/2 cup	3/4 cup
3. Bread and bread alternates (whole grain or enriched):			
Bread	1/2 slice	1/2 slice	1 slice
or cornbread, rolls, muffins, or biscuits	1/2 serving	1/2 serving	1 serving
or cold dry cereal (volume or weight, whichever is less)	1/4 cup or 1/3 oz.	1/3 cup or 1/2 oz.	3/4 cup or 1 oz.
or cooked cereal, pasta, noodle products, or cereal grains	1/4 cup	1/4 cup	1/2 cup
4. Meat or meat alternates	1/2 oz.	1/2 oz.	1 oz.
Lean meat, fish, or poultry (edible portion as served)			
or cheese	1/2 oz.	1/2 oz.	1 oz.
or egg	1/2 egg	1/2 egg	1 egg
or cooked dry beans or peas[1]	1/8 cup	1/8 cup	1/4 cup
or peanut butter, soynut butter, or other nut or seed butters	1 Tbsp.	1 Tbsp.	2 Tbsps.
or peanuts, soy nuts, tree nuts, or seeds[2]	1/2 oz.	1/2 oz.	1 oz.
or yogurt	1/4 cup	1/4 cup	1/2 cup
or an equivalent quantity of any combination of the above meat/meat alternates.			

[1]In the same meal service, dried beans or dried peas may be used as a meat alternate or as a vegetable; however, such use does not satisfy the requirement for both components.

[2]Tree nuts and seeds that may be used as meat alternates are listed in Section 1 of the CCFP Guidelines.

[3]No more than 50 percent of the requirement shall be met with nuts or seeds. Nuts *or* seeds shall be combined with another meat/meat alternate to fulfill the requirement. For the purpose of determining combinations, 1 oz. of nuts or seeds is equal to 1 oz. of cooked lean meat, poultry, or fish.

[4]Juice may not be served when milk is served as the only other component.

Modifying Foods for Children of Different Ages

It may be necessary for you to adjust recipes, including those in this book, to make foods suitable for children at different levels of development. You may also need to modify the form of simple foods like apples or toast.

One reason for this is that the texture or shape of a certain food may make it difficult for a very young child to eat it. You want her to be able to get the food into her mouth, chew it, and swallow it without frustration, because, after all, she should feel successful and happy about her eating experiences. You also want her to get the benefit of its nutritional contribution, which she won't if she gives up on it.

Another important reason for modifying some of the foods you serve is that young children are much more likely to choke on foods that are generally safe for older children. Lastly, certain food ingredients are unsuitable for infants.

❏ Never feed honey to a child less than one year of age; this precaution is necessary to avoid the danger of infant botulism.[3]

❏ Avoid adding salt and sugar to the foods you serve infants.

❏ Minimize choking hazards for children younger than four years old:[4]

- Chop nuts and seeds finely.

- Slice grapes in half lengthwise.

- Slice hot dogs in quarters lengthwise.

- Shred hard raw vegetables and fruits.

- Remove pits from cherries, plums, peaches, etc.

- Remove bones from fish.

- Spread peanut butter thinly.

- Avoid giving young children popcorn and hard candies at all.

❏ Depending upon an infant's age and eating ability, you can puree, mash, or chop many of the same foods you are feeding to older children (if you will be adding sugar, salt, or heavy seasonings to these foods, remove the infant's portion first).

❑ Young children prefer meat that is very tender: cooking with moist heat and chopping or shredding the meat finely, or using ground poultry or beef, will make it easier for children to eat.

❑ Remember that toddlers and preschoolers enjoy "finger foods."

❑ Some young children prefer foods that are prepared simply and singly. They may balk at tuna salad sandwiches but eat plain flaked tuna and bread wedges eagerly, or they may enjoy plain steamed carrots and reject carrots mixed into a casserole.

Following the Dietary Guidelines the Yummy Way

It's possible to eat the recommended number of servings from each of the basic food groups and still be poorly nourished. This commonly happens when the foods chosen are high in fat, sugar, or salt, if the foods are limited in their variety, or if foods have been stored or prepared in ways that cause losses of nutrients.

Several health organizations have made recommendations for healthful diets that address these concerns. One such set of recommendations is the **Dietary Guidelines for Americans,** issued jointly by the U.S. Department of Agriculture and the Department of Health and Human Services in 1990. The Dietary Guidelines don't give us hard numbers, but they steer us in the right direction.

Dietary Guidelines for Americans[2]

- Eat a variety of foods.
- Maintain healthy weight.
- Choose a diet low in fat, saturated fat, and cholesterol.
- Choose a diet with plenty of vegetables, fruits, and grain products.
- Use sugars only in moderation.
- Use salt and sodium only in moderation.
- If you drink alcoholic beverages, do so in moderation.

It's possible to follow the Dietary Guidelines and still have a lot of fun eating (and cooking). Some foods may need to show up on the menu less often or in smaller amounts, or some of your favorite recipes may need adjustments. Be patient, proceed with an attitude of experimentation, and realize that it may take a little while for jaded taste buds to get used to the changes. Some day you may be surprised to find that soups you ate for years just taste too salty. In the next few pages, we are going to show you how to put more variety into your menus, cut down on fat, sugar, and sodium (salt), and add more fiber and complex carbohydrates from fruits, vegetables, and grains.

Variety Brings Your Menus to Life

Variety helps make your meals more interesting and more nutritious. A good start is remembering to serve foods from the four main food groups every day. The next step is to beware of getting into ruts when planning menus (don't worry, we all get into them). Sometimes we have to curl up with a good cookbook, stroll through the produce department at our local market, or try out a new (perhaps ethnic) restaurant to find inspiration. We love doing that sort of research!

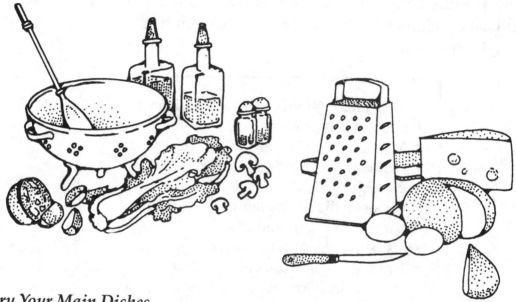

Vary Your Main Dishes . . .

- Look at your choices! You needn't serve chicken 3 times a week when you can choose from dried beans, peas, lentils, peanut butter, cheese, eggs, fish, other seafood, turkey, beef, pork, and lamb . . .
- Balance meat dishes with vegetarian entrees.
- Try some ethnic recipes.
- Try a main-dish salad.

Tired of Carrot and Celery Sticks? Try These Vegetables Raw Instead:

- tomatoes
- cucumbers
- sugar-snap peas
- green or red peppers
- jicama
- cauliflower
- asparagus (best blanched)
- snow peas (also best blanched)
- turnips
- fennel
- cabbage
- sprouts
- summer squashes
- broccoli
- radishes
- mushrooms

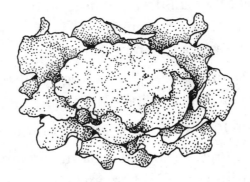

Grain Products Besides Cold Cereal You Can Serve at Breakfast:

- hot cereals (oatmeal, whole wheat varieties, grits, brown rice, polenta)
- tortillas
- muffins, quick breads
- pancakes, waffles, french toast
- sandwiches
- pizza
- rice cakes, graham crackers
- Swiss Breakfast (page 107)
- bagels, pita bread, cornbread
- noodle kugel

First, Let's Ditch Some Fat

❏ Choose lean meats, fish, poultry, lower-fat cheeses, and, especially, dried beans as protein sources. Try combining small amounts of high-fat protein foods like ground beef or cheese with cooked dried beans (example: chili with beans).

❏ Portion sizes of meats should be small.

❏ Broil, bake, or steam foods rather than frying them.

❏ Trim the fat from meat and take the skin off poultry. Drain cooked ground beef before adding to other ingredients.

❏ Don't automatically add fat such as butter to breads, grains, and vegetables. Let children get used to the taste of foods without it. Many children enjoy salads more without dressing; that's a nice habit to get into!

❏ Limit your use of whole eggs. Two egg whites can fill in for one whole egg in most recipes.

❏ Read labels on food packaging and opt for low-fat products.

❏ Use non-fat or low-fat milk in cooking. Evaporated skim milk is a good substitute for light cream.

❏ Use yogurt as a substitute for mayonnaise or sour cream.

❏ Experiment with cutting the amount of fat in your favorite recipes. It's amazing what you can do with a tablespoon of oil rather than a half-cup.

Helpful Hint

How to Remove More of the Fat from Ground Beef

Cook the meat and drain off all the fat you can. Cover with cold water and refrigerate overnight. The next day, you can skim off the fat that has congealed, drain the meat, and use it in your recipe.

- ❏ Avoid prebreaded meat items.

- ❏ Use nonstick or seasoned cast-iron skillets.

- ❏ Limit your use of butter, cream, whole milk, most cheeses, hard margarine, shortening, lard, coconut and palm oils, and foods containing them.

- ❏ Use olive or canola oil in place of butter or margarine where practical. Oil cannot be directly substituted for butter or shortening in baked goods without changing their texture. There are many recipes available for bakery items with a minimum of fat and saturated fat, however (see *Appendix D— Resources* in the back of this book).

- ❏ Serve high-fat foods in smaller portions and less often.

- ❏ ***Do not restrict fat in the diets of children under the age of two.***

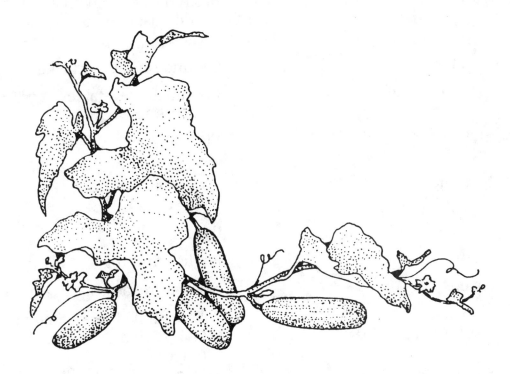

High-Fat Foods	Lower-Fat Alternatives
Whole milk	Non-fat or low-fat milk
Sour cream	Yogurt, light sour cream
Hard cheeses—Cheddar, swiss, jack, American	Reduced-fat cheeses, low-fat cottage cheese
Cream soups (made with cream or cream sauce)	Clear soups or "cream" soups made with evaporated skim milk or vegetable purees
Mayonnaise	Yogurt, reduced-fat mayonnaise, mustard
Luncheon meats and sausages	Turkey and chicken breast, lean ham, lean roast beef
Oil-packed tuna	Water-packed tuna
Snack chips (potato, corn)	Toast points, **Pita Points** (page 108) pretzels, rice cakes
Gravies	Broth thickened with a little flour or cornstarch, tomato sauce, catsup
Ground beef	Ground turkey or chicken
Pizza with sausage	Pizza with vegetables or plain cheese
Vegetables frozen with butter sauce	Plain frozen vegetables
Pastries and cakes	Lower-fat muffins and quick breads
Doughnuts	Bagels
Croissants	English muffins
Ice cream	Non-fat frozen yogurt, sorbet
Fried foods French fried potatoes	Baked, broiled, or steamed foods **Oven Fried Potato Sticks** (page 94)
Fried fish	**Homemade Fish Sticks** (page 87)
Chicken nuggets	**Chicken Fingers** (page 89)
Buttered popcorn	Air-popped popcorn
Sugar cookies, sandwich cookies	Graham crackers, Fig Newtons®

Next, Let's Get Rid of Some Sugar

❏ Watch out for "hidden sugar" in convenience foods. Read labels!!! Sugar = sucrose, glucose, dextrose, invert sugar, fructose, corn syrup, corn sweeteners, maple syrup, honey, molasses, raw sugar, turbinado sugar, Sucanat . . .

❏ Keep the sugar bowl and honey bear off the table.

❏ Serve fresh fruits, unsweetened frozen fruits, or fruits canned in natural juices or water.

❏ Serve 100% fruit juices instead of fruit drinks. Read labels carefully!

❏ Check the breakfast cereals you're using; they should have less than 6 grams of sugar per serving.

❏ Sweeten cold or hot cereals with fruit, like bananas.

❏ Experiment with cutting back the sugar (up to 50%) in your recipes.

❏ Serve muffins instead of cupcakes, graham crackers instead of cookies (or make your own cookies with less sugar).

❏ Use vanilla, cinnamon, nutmeg, or allspice to enhance sweet flavors.

❏ Add your own fruit to plain yogurt rather than buy the sweetened variety. Mash it first, and it won't seem so tart.

❏ When you do serve foods high in sugar, use small portions and serve them less often.

Foods High in Sugar	
chocolate milk	canned fruits in syrup
milkshakes	flavored gelatin desserts
soft drinks	candies
fruit drinks/ades	sweetened coconut
jam, jellies	flavored yogurts
syrups, sweet sauce	puddings
ice cream, sherbet	sweet pickle relish
pies, pastries	many children's cereals
cakes, cookies	sweet rolls, doughnuts

Kids Don't Need All That Salt, Either

Foods High in Salt (aka Sodium)

Soy sauce	Bouillon
Gravies	MSG
Pickles	Olives
Sauerkraut	Commercial salad dressings
Bacon	Ham
Frankfurters	Bologna
Canned meats	Sausage
Corned beef	Processed cheeses
Salted nuts/	Salted crackers
nut butters	Many prepared foods
Snack chips	Miso
Canned soups	

❑ Don't add salt to pasta, rice, cereals, and vegetable cooking water.

❑ Leave the salt shaker and soy sauce bottle off the table.

❑ *Gradually* reduce the amount of salt in your recipes. Never add salt to baby foods.

❑ Use chicken or vegetable stock or water instead of bouillon.

❑ Use herbs, spices, and lemon juice to enhance the flavors of foods.

❑ Use unsalted nut butters and crackers with less salt.

❑ Serve high-sodium foods less often and in smaller quantities.

❑ Make homemade versions of foods you usually buy ready-to-serve or as mixes.

❑ Read labels! Check the nutrition information for the milligrams of sodium in a serving.

Now There's Room for More Starch and Fiber

❏ Serve more bread, potatoes, tortillas, rice, pasta, and unsweetened cereals, and fewer cookies, pastries, doughnuts, and sweetened cereals.

❏ Look for *whole grain* cereal products, breads, and tortillas.

❏ Serve lots of fruits and vegetables, *unpeeled.*

❏ Serve *raw* fruits and vegetables often.

❏ Serve (cooked) dried beans and peas often.

❏ Serve dried fruits like prunes, raisins or dried apricots occasionally; they are sticky, however, so make sure children brush their teeth afterwards.

❏ Make sure children drink plenty of water so the fiber can move through their intestines.

❏ Don't depend on bran products to add fiber to children's diets; they generally don't need them.

High Fiber Foods

Whole grain breads	Popcorn
Shredded wheat cereals	Dried beans, lentils
Nutrigrain® cereals	Fresh fruits with
Oatmeal	skins
Brown rice	Berries
Bulgur wheat	Bananas
Millet	Dried fruits
Nuts and seeds	Raw vegetables

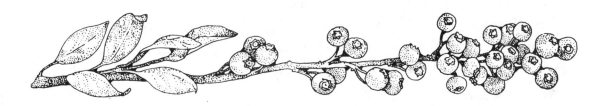

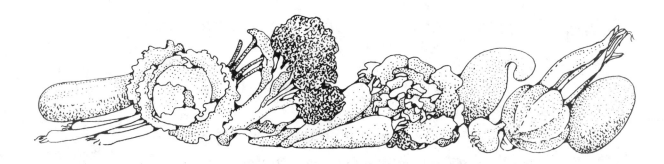

Foods Chock-Full of Vitamin A

Vitamin A is found in enormous quantities in fish liver oils and in animal livers in general. Milk products, butter, and margarine are also good sources of vitamin A.

What end up being the most significant sources of vitamin A in our diets, however, are fruits and vegetables. Actually, they contain a form of vitamin A called *carotene*, which is getting a lot of favorable press lately for its possible role in preventing cancer, and is basically harmless even when eaten in huge amounts. So plan to serve some of these fruits and vegetables at least four times a week![5]

Vegetables

Asparagus
Broccoli
Carrots
Chard
Chili peppers
Collard greens
Dandelion greens
Kale
Mixed vegetables (frozen)

Mustard greens
Peppers (sweet red)
Pumpkin
Spinach
Squash, winter
Sweet potatoes
Tomatoes
Turnip greens

Fruits

Apricots
Cantaloupe
Cherries (red sour)
Mangoes
Nectarines

Papayas
Peaches (except canned)
Plums (canned purple)
Prunes

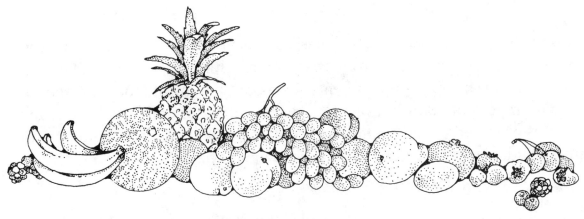

Foods Bursting With Vitamin C!

Foods containing vitamin C should be included in meals every day. Since vitamin C can be destroyed by cooking and exposure to air, you must take special care with these foods. Serve fruits and vegetables raw or lightly cooked to get the most vitamin C from them.

Vegetables

Asparagus
Broccoli
Brussels sprouts
Cabbage
Cauliflower
Chili peppers
Collards
Cress, garden
Dandelion greens
Kale

Mustard greens
Okra
Peppers, red and green
Potatoes
Spinach
Sweet potatoes
Tomatoes
Turnip greens
Turnips

Fruits

Cantaloupe
Grapefruit
Grapefruit juice
Guavas
Honeydew melon
Lemons
Mangoes

Oranges
Orange juice
Papayas
Raspberries
Strawberries
Tangerines
Tangelos

Good Sources of Iron

Iron is one nutrient that often comes up short in children's diets. The iron found in meats ("heme" iron) is absorbed much more efficiently than that from non-meat sources ("non-heme" iron), but non-meat foods can and do make important contributions to the iron intake of children. Non-heme iron is absorbed better if vitamin C-containing foods are eaten along with it. Include several sources of iron in your menus daily.[5]

Meat and Meat Alternatives Group

Dried beans and peas   Peanut butter
Eggs   Shellfish
Meats, especially liver   Turkey

Vegetables

Asparagus (canned)   Parsnips
Beans (green, lima, canned)   Peas
Beet greens   Spinach
Beets (canned)   Squash, winter
Broccoli   Sweet potatoes
Brussels sprouts   Tomato juice
Chard   Tomato paste
Collards   Tomato puree
Kale   Tomatoes (canned)
Mustard greens   Turnip greens
Parsley

Fruits

Apples (dried)   Peaches (dried)
Apricots (canned or dried)   Prunes
Cherries (canned)   Raisins
Dates   Strawberries
Figs (dried)   Watermelon
Grapes (canned)

Breads and Grain Products

Any enriched or whole-grain breads and cereals

Your Faithful Lunchbox Guide

Protein-Rich Foods

Roasted chicken breast (1–2 oz)
Lean roast beef (1–2 oz)
Roasted turkey (1–2 oz)
Tuna or leftover fish (1–2 oz)
Hardboiled egg (1)
Peanut butter (2 T)
Lowfat cheese (1–2 oz)
Lowfat cottage cheese (3/8 c)
Tofu cubes (3–4 oz)
Tempeh "fingers" (2 oz)
Beans, bean soups (1/2 c)
Salmon loaf / patty (2 oz)
Veggie-burger

Calcium-Rich Foods

Lowfat or nonfat milk (6 oz)
Yogurt (3/4 c)
Lowfat cheeses (1 oz)
Tofu* (5 oz)
Cottage cheese (3/4 c)
Corn tortillas (2)

*Must contain calcium sulfate, not nigari

Starchy Foods

Bread (1 slice, small roll)
Bagel (1/2)
Flour or corn tortilla (1)
Rice or pasta (1/3–1/2 c)
Crackers (3–4)
Rice cakes (2, or 6–8 mini)
Unsweetened cereal (1/2 c)
Muffin, small
Tabouli (1/2 c)
Bread sticks

Fruits and Vegetables

Carrot sticks
Celery "boats"
Zucchini sticks
Turnip rounds
Jicama slices
Broccoli "trees"
Sprouts
Tomatoes
Lettuce
Pepper rings or sticks
Apples, oranges, pears, berries, bananas, kiwi slices, pineapple . . .
Unsweetened juices

DO use leftovers and combination foods: casseroles, salads, dips made from cottage cheese or yogurt, soups. . . . See how your child likes cold leftover enchiladas at home first, though!

Snacks Are Important

Snacks can make important contributions to good nutrition. Children often can't eat enough to satisfy all of their needs at the standard three meals, and they may feel tired and miserable when opportunities to eat are spaced too far apart (so can adults, actually). The keys to making snacks work are *timing* and *food choices.*

❑ Establish regular snack times. Don't give handouts all day long and don't let the children fill up on juice when they're thirsty.

❑ Schedule snacks a few hours before the next meal (so the children will be hungry enough at mealtime to eat, but not so hungry they are frantic), and a few hours after the last meal (so the children don't get the idea that they can refuse a meal and be rescued shortly thereafter).

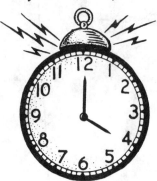

❑ Snacks can be fairly substantial if it will be a long time before the children will eat again—lighter if you just need to hold off the hunger for a little while. When children are in child care for long afternoons, they may need a second, light snack around five o'clock. Parents facing the ride home and preparing late dinners are usually very appreciative when their children are fortified and reasonably cheerful!

❑ Be creative! Snacktime is a wonderful opportunity to use up leftovers, serve foods that are new and unusual, and have the kids participate in food preparation.

❑ Avoid serving foods that are highly sweetened or salted; make what you offer as nutritious as possible.

Snacktime Mix and Match

Plan snacks to include a serving from at least *two* of the four food groups. Be creative! Here are some ideas to get you started . . .

Bread/Cereal Group

Pita Points (page 108)
Rice cakes
Bagels
Graham crackers
Quick breads and muffins
Savory Scrambled Cereals
    (page 112)
Nori-Maki Rolls (page 109)
Tortillas
Toast fingers
Pancakes
Bread sticks
Cold cereal
English muffins

Meat and Meat Alternatives

Vegetarian chili (canned or
    homemade, page 86)
Bean or lentil soups
Hummous (page 112)
Cheese (preferably reduced-fat
    varieties)
Cottage cheese
Turkey loaf cubes
Yogurt
Peanut butter
Mock Sour Cream (page 110)
    as a dip or topping
Tuna salad
Bean Dip (page 111)

Fruit & Vegetable Group

Micro-Fruit (page 100)
Any fresh fruit
Any raw vegetable
Vegetable soups
Soft-Serve Fruit (page 101)
Wiggly Fruit (page 100)
Unsweetened canned
    or frozen fruit
Baked potatoes or *Oven Fried
    Potato Sticks* (page 94)
Unsweetened fruit juice

Milk Group*

Fluid milk
Milk in "shakes" or smoothies

*Only fluid milk is in this group for
Child Care Food Program
reimbursement purposes, though
cheese, cottage cheese, and yogurt
are also considered dairy foods.

How Does Your Menu Measure Up?

A good menu does more than meet the basic requirements for servings from the Four Food Groups. With proper planning, you can make sure that the foods you serve are appealing, emphasize critical nutrients, and teach healthful eating habits. You will also be able to manage your costs and workflow better. Check your menu against the criteria below:

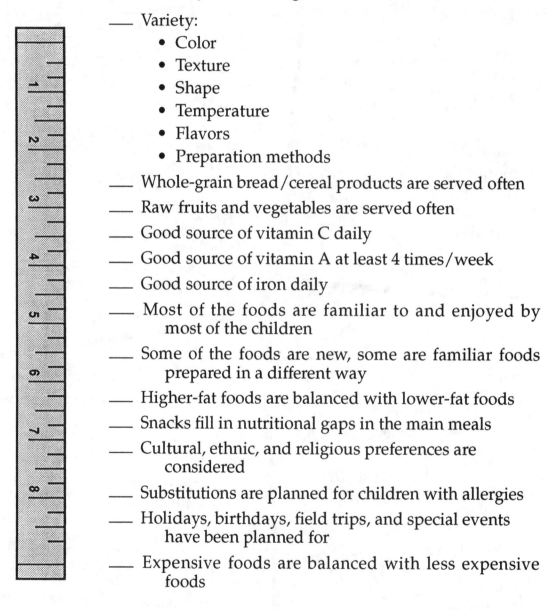

— Variety:
  - Color
  - Texture
  - Shape
  - Temperature
  - Flavors
  - Preparation methods

— Whole-grain bread/cereal products are served often

— Raw fruits and vegetables are served often

— Good source of vitamin C daily

— Good source of vitamin A at least 4 times/week

— Good source of iron daily

— Most of the foods are familiar to and enjoyed by most of the children

— Some of the foods are new, some are familiar foods prepared in a different way

— Higher-fat foods are balanced with lower-fat foods

— Snacks fill in nutritional gaps in the main meals

— Cultural, ethnic, and religious preferences are considered

— Substitutions are planned for children with allergies

— Holidays, birthdays, field trips, and special events have been planned for

— Expensive foods are balanced with less expensive foods

Computers and Your Kitchen

What do computers have to do with feeding kids? Well, you can use a computer to plan menus, adjust and store recipes, generate a shopping list, and perform various accounting functions. You can also use a computer to determine what levels of nutrients your menus are providing.

There are many computer programs available that will analyze individual foods, recipes, or a day's menus for nutrient content. They also compare a given menu with the Recommended Dietary Allowances (RDA) for persons of a specified age, sex, and size. They can also compute the percentage of fat and the amounts of sugar, cholesterol, and fiber in foods and meals. Two such programs, *DINE* for the Macintosh and *Nutrition Wizard* for IBM-compatible computers, are simple to use and available through:

> **Center for Science in the Public Interest** (CSPI)
> 1875 Connecticut Avenue, NW, #300
> Washington DC 20009
> (202) 667-7483
>
> **DINE,** $219.95 (hard drive required)
> **Nutrition Wizard,** $99.95 (specify 5 1/4" or 3 1/2" disk size)

If you aren't inclined to use the computer yourself, perhaps you have a friend who would love an excuse to work with a new program. You can also seek out a Registered Dietitian (check your Yellow Pages) who may be willing to perform menu analyses for you.

CHAPTER FOUR

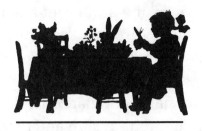

The Recipes

About the Recipes . . .

In developing these recipes, we kept in mind that people who take care of children generally don't have a lot of time to cook. Even people who cook for children as a full-time job enjoy saving time! What we are promoting is the use of simple foods, made "from scratch." These foods are usually cheaper and taste fresher than processed foods. And very importantly, they give us more control over the amounts of fat, sugar, salt, and additives we serve.

Most of the recipes have been tested in very large quantities as well as very small. We aimed for testers in a variety of situations and in different parts of the country to make sure that we got a good picture of taste preferences and that ingredients would be readily available. There are some recipes that will obviously be unworkable due to time, transportation, or storage problems if you are running a centralized kitchen serving 500 children. They may, however, be useful as cooking projects in classrooms.

We have cut the fat, salt, and sugar in these recipes as much as possible, while still pleasing our obliging "taste testers," both children and adults. You may find that they don't taste salty or sweet enough, but as your (and the children's) taste buds get used to less salt and sugar, they'll be fine. We also made the foods less spicy than we would ordinarily serve to adults. If you know that the children you're cooking for are very sensitive to spicy foods, you may want to cut the seasoning even further. On the other hand, some children have quite adventuresome palates, and you can be a little freer with the chili powder and such.

The serving sizes listed are the minimum amounts that must be served to count for reimbursement through the Child Care Food Program or School Lunch Program.* You will want to make large enough quantities to allow for second helpings, and you are probably aware, by now, of which items are likely to be especially popular with the children you're cooking for. In the interest of the children's health and of your budget, however, we don't suggest that you feel obliged to serve huge amounts of the meat or meat substitutes. Protein-rich foods (except dried beans) are usually the most expensive, and children don't need as much as you may think. If the children are still hungry, they can eat more vegetables, fruits, and grains instead. It's a habit that will serve them well when they grow up!

Bon Appetit!

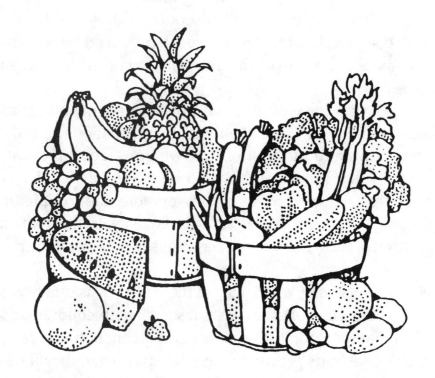

*Unless otherwise specified, 1 serving of vegetables or fruit = 1/4 cup

The Recipes

Lentil Soup
"Gentle Lentil Soup"

2 1/2 cups lentils, rinsed and
  drained
7 cups water or stock
2 medium onions, chopped
3 cloves garlic, minced
juice of one lemon
salt and pepper to taste

2 stalks celery, chopped
2 T. olive oil
1 or 2 bunches spinach, chard, or
  collards, washed and chopped
  coarsely

1. Sauté onions, garlic and celery in the olive oil, 5–10 minutes.
2. Add lentils, and water or stock and simmer until lentils are very soft. If necessary, add more water to get soup to desired consistency.
3. Add greens, salt and pepper. Simmer for 10 more minutes or until greens are tender.
4. Stir in lemon juice right before serving.

Serves 16 preschool or 12 school-age children
1 meat alternative

❑ ❑ ❑

Garbo-Burgers
"Beanie Burgers"

1 15-1/2 oz. can garbanzo beans,
  drained
1 1/3 cup rolled oats
1 cup water
1 t. Italian seasoning

1 small onion, minced or
  1 t. onion powder
1/8 t. garlic powder
1 1/2 T. soy sauce or
  2 t. Worchestershire sauce
1 T. olive oil

1. Run beans through food processor until they have a texture like ground meat.
2. Add remaining ingredients (except for oil) and allow to sit for 10–15 minutes so water is absorbed.
3. Heat olive oil in skillet.
4. Spoon large or small patties into the skillet, press down into burger shapes.
5. Cook on both sides until browned.

Note: Use as burgers or to fill in for the veal in a vegetarian version of "Veal Parmesan." Small patties can be eaten as finger food and/or dipped into sauces, too.

Serves 4–5 preschool or 3 school-age children
1 meat alternative

White Bean Soup*
"Speckled Soup"

1 1/2 cups white beans
4 cups water or stock
2 cloves garlic, minced
2 stalks celery, chopped
2 carrots, chopped
1 onion, chopped
2 T. olive oil

1 T. dried basil
1/2 lb. green beans in 1" pieces,
   or 1/2 lb. zucchini, sliced in
   half-moons
2 T. lemon juice
3/4 t. salt
pepper to taste

1. Soak beans in water to cover by 2" overnight. Drain in the morning.
2. Sauté garlic, onion, celery, and carrots in oil for about 10 minutes.
3. Add soaked beans and the 4 cups of water or stock.
4. Simmer until beans are tender, about 45 minutes.
5. Add basil and green beans or zucchini and simmer another 30 minutes or so, until tender.
6. Before serving, stir in lemon juice, salt and pepper.

Serves 8 preschool or 6 school-age children
1 meat alternative

❏ ❏ ❏

Easier-Than-Lasagna

8 oz. macaroni or spiral pasta
1 onion, chopped
4 cloves garlic, chopped
2 T. olive oil
2 t. oregano
1 t. basil
1 bay leaf

1 28-oz. can (3 3/4 c.) crushed
   tomatoes
1 t. salt
1/2 cup water
2 cups cottage or ricotta cheese
1/2 cup Parmesan cheese
9 oz. brick or jack cheese, grated

1. Sauté onion and garlic in the oil.
2. Add tomatoes, herbs, salt and water and simmer 30 minutes.
3. Cook pasta until just tender.
4. Stir all ingredients together except the brick or jack cheese to sprinkle on top. Bake for 20 minutes at 375°.

Serves 12 preschool or 8 school-age children
1 meat + 1 bread/grain + 1 vegetable

*Adapted from *Still Life with Menu* © 1988 by Mollie Katzen. Reprinted by permission of Ten Speed Press, Berkeley, California.

Chilaquiles*

1 dozen corn tortillas,
   several days old
1 cup onions, chopped
2 cloves garlic, pressed or
   1/4 t. garlic powder
2 t. chili powder

1 t. cumin powder
1 1/2 cups lowfat cottage cheese
1 1/2 cups canned crushed tomatoes
6 oz. grated jack or Cheddar cheese
salt to taste
1 T. oil

1. Cut tortillas into wedges or tear into strips.
2. Sauté onions in oil for 5 minutes. (A non-stick or cast iron skillet that's ovenproof is ideal for this.)
3. Add tortilla pieces, chili powder, garlic, cumin and salt.
4. Toss until the tortilla pieces are wilted.
5. Pureé cottage cheese and tomatoes in blender until smooth.
6. Stir gently into tortilla pieces.
7. Sprinkle with grated cheese.
8. Bake at 350° for about 20 minutes.

Serves 8 preschool or 6 school-age children
1 meat alternative + 1 bread/grain

❏ ❏ ❏

One-Pot Macaroni and Cheese

8 oz. dry macaroni or other pasta
2 cups lowfat milk
1 1/2 T. cornstarch
3/4 t. salt
1/4 t. fresh-ground pepper

1/2 t. dry mustard
1/4 t. paprika
12 oz. sharp Cheddar cheese, grated
2 scallions, green part only, thinly
   sliced or 2 T. minced chives
   (optional)

1. Cook macaroni.
2. While macaroni is cooking, combine milk and dry ingredients in a jar and shake very well.
3. When macaroni is tender, drain it and return to pan.
4. Add milk mixture and stir gently over medium heat until sauce thickens.
5. Add cheese and optional scallions or chives, stir until melted, and serve.

Serves 8 preschool or 6 school-age children
1 meat alternative + 1 bread/grain

*Adapted from *Laurel's Kitchen* by Laurel Robertson, Carol Flinders, and Bronwen Godfrey. Petaluma, CA: Nilgiri Press, 1976.

Vegetarian Chili
"Jack & Jilli Chili"

3 1-lb. cans of pinto or black beans, drained (save liquid)
1 T. oil
1 large onion, chopped
1 bell pepper, chopped

3 garlic cloves, chopped
1 t. cumin
2 t. chili powder
1 1-lb. can of tomatoes
1/2 t. salt

1. Sauté onion and green pepper in oil for about 5 minutes.
2. Add garlic and sauté another minute.
3. Add remaining ingredients and simmer about 20–30 minutes. Add bean liquid if necessary to retain moist consistency.

Variation: *Chili-Mac:* Toss with 6–8 ounces of macaroni, cooked.

Serves 12 pre-school or 9 school-age children

1 meat alternative (+ 1 bread/grain if macaroni is added)

❑ ❑ ❑

Tuna Salad
"Looney Tooney Salad"

2 6 1/2-oz. cans water-packed tuna, drained and flaked
1/2 cup plain yogurt or a mixture of 1/2 yogurt and 1/2 mayonnaise
2 minced scallions

2 minced celery ribs
1/2 t. curry powder
1/4 t. salt
4 T. water chestnuts, chopped (optional)

1. Mix all ingredients together.
2. Eat as salad or sandwich spread.

Serves 7 preschool or 5 school-age children

1 meat

Yummy-for-the-Tummy Baked Fish

1 lb. fish filets (flounder, sole,
perch, orange roughy)
2 1/2 cups fresh whole wheat
bread crumbs
1/3 cup chopped onion
1 1/2 T. lemon juice
1/2 t. Italian seasoning

1 t. parsley flakes
1/4 t. salt
1/8 t. pepper
1 T. olive oil
3 T. Parmesan cheese
1/8 t. garlic powder

1. Spread out fish filets in oiled baking pan.
2. Combine remaining ingredients and spread over fish.
3. Bake at 400° for about 15 minutes or at 375° for 20 minutes.

Serves 7 preschool or 5 school-age children

1 meat

❑　❑　❑

Homemade Fish Sticks
"Sea Sticks"

1 lb. snapper or cod, cut into sticks
1 egg white, beaten
1 1/2 T. oil
3/4 cup corn flake crumbs
1/2 t. onion powder
1/16 t. garlic powder
salt and pepper to taste

1. Mix together beaten egg white and oil.
2. Combine cereal crumbs, onion powder, garlic power, salt and pepper.
3. Dip fish sticks into egg white mixture, then roll in seasoned flakes.
4. Bake at 400°, 10–15 minutes, turning once.

Serves 7 preschool or 5 school-age children

1 meat

Chow Mein Salad

1/2 lb. Napa (Chinese) cabbage,
    shredded
1/3 lb. mung bean sprouts
1/4 lb. snow peas
1–2 scallions, tops only, thinly sliced

1 rib celery, thinly sliced
1 8 oz. can water chestnuts, sliced
9 oz. cooked chicken meat, shredded
1 5-oz. can chow mein noodles,
    (crispy type)

Dressing

2 T. plain rice vinegar
2 T. toasted sesame oil
1 T. vegetable oil
2 T. soy sauce

1 garlic clove, pressed or
    1/8 t. garlic powder
1/2 t. powdered ginger
1/2 t. sugar

1. Blanch bean sprouts and snow peas separately, about 2 minutes, in boiling water. Let cool in refrigerator.
2. Combine all salad ingredients in large bowl.
3. Combine dressing ingredients and toss with salad.

Variations: Romaine lettuce can be use instead of Napa cabbage. You can substitute 9 oz. of cooked shrimp for the chicken.

Serves 6 preschool or 4 school-age children

1 meat + 2 vegetables

❏ ❏ ❏

Marek's Chicken

4 lbs. chicken pieces
2 cloves garlic, pressed
juice of one lemon
1" piece of ginger root
    peeled and chopped fine

2 bunches scallions, cut into
    1" pieces
1 T. curry powder
2 T. oil
salt to taste

1. Remove skin from chicken pieces.
2. Brown chicken and ginger in oil, about 5 minutes.
3. Add scallions, garlic and curry powder and sauté about another 5 minutes.
4. Add the lemon juice, about 1/4 cup water, and salt. Cover the pan and simmer until the chicken is thoroughly cooked, adding more water if necessary to keep the mixture very moist. Serve with rice.

Note: Chris's friend, Marek, learned to cook this dish in Nepal.

Serves 16 preschool or 12 school-age children

1 meat

Chicken Fingers
"Slim Pickin' Chicken Fingers"

1 lb. boneless, skinless chicken breasts sliced across the "grain" in 3/4" strips

1 cup corn flake crumbs (ready-made crumbs are cheaper than the cereal!)

1 1/4 t. Spike seasoning
1/8 t. garlic powder
1/8 t. pepper
2 egg whites
1 T. oil

1. Combine cereal crumbs and seasonings.
2. Beat oil into egg whites.
3. Roll chicken pieces in egg mixture, then in crumbs.
4. Spread out on a greased baking sheet.
5. Bake at 400° for 15 minutes.

Variation: For eggless version, roll chicken pieces in 1/2 cup yogurt thinned with 1 T. milk, then in crumbs.

Serves 6 preschool or 4 school-age children

1 meat

Three Marinades for Chicken
(chicken pieces or strips of chicken breast)

Mustard-Honey Marinade

1/4 cup honey
2 T. Dijon-type mustard
1 clove garlic, pressed, or 1/8 t. garlic powder
2 T. rice vinegar
1 1/2 t. dark sesame oil
1 1/2 T. soy sauce

Mint-Garlic Marinade

1 cup plain yogurt
2 T. chopped onion
1 t. dried mint
2 cloves garlic, pressed, or 1/4 t. garlic powder
1/2 t. salt

Teriyaki Marinade

1/4 cup soy sauce
1/4 cup orange juice
1 T. brown sugar
2 cloves fresh garlic, pressed, or 1/4 t. garlic powder
1 t. fresh grated ginger, or 1/2 t. powdered ginger

Each recipe marinates about 2 lbs. of chicken

Sloppy Josephines

1 lb. ground turkey
3/4 cup onion, chopped
1 cup tomato sauce
2 T. prepared mustar
1 T. Worchestershire sauce

1 t. brown sugar
1/8 t. garlic powder
salt and pepper to taste
whole grain hot dog or
   hamburger buns

1. Sauté onion and turkey gently until turkey is cooked through, breaking up large clumps. Add small amount of oil if necessary to prevent sticking.
2. Add remaining ingredients and simmer 15 minutes.
3. Serve on hot dog or hamburger buns.

Serves 7 preschool or 5 school-age children
1 meat + 1 bread/grain

❑ ❑ ❑

Turkey Loaf
"Loafin' Turkey"

1 lb. ground turkey
1 10-oz. package frozen broccoli
1 cup sharp Cheddar cheese, grated
1 cup soft bread crumbs
1 egg

1/3 cup milk
1/2 cup chopped onion
1 t. fines herbes
2 t. prepared mustard
1/2 t. salt
1/8 t. pepper

1. Steam broccoli until just barely cooked.
2. Mix with all other ingredients in a large bowl.
3. Pack into a loaf pan and bake about 1 hour at 350°.

Serves 9 preschool or 6 school-age children
1 meat

Taco Salad

8 cups shredded lettuce
1 lb. fresh tomatoes, diced
6 oz. cooked chicken or turkey,
    shredded or diced or
    6 oz. cooked ground beef or
    1 1/2 cups cooked dried beans
    (kidney, pinto, or black beans)

6 oz. grated Cheddar or jack cheese
1 cup crumbled tortilla chips

Dressing

3 T. oil
1 1/2 T. red wine vinegar
2 T. water
1/8 t. garlic powder

1/2 t. oregano
1/2 t. chili powder
1/4 t. cumin powder
1/4 t. salt

1. Combine dressing ingredients.
2. Toss lettuce and tomatoes with dressing.
3. Spread meat or beans and cheese over top.
4. Sprinkle crumbled tortilla chips over all.

Optional additions: fresh raw corn cut from the cob, scallions, cilantro, avocado.

Serves 8 preschool or 6 school-age children
1 meat + 2 vegetables

Salmon Cakes or Muffins

1 1-lb. can of salmon, flaked
1/2 cup chopped onion
2 T. lemon juice
1 1/2 t. dill weed
1/4 t. tabasco or dash of
  cayenne pepper

3/4 cup cracker meal
2 egg whites
1/2 cup milk
1/4 t. salt
1/4 t. pepper

1. Mix all ingredients well.
2. Shape into patties and place on a greased baking sheet or portion into greased muffin cups.
3. Bake at 400° for about 20 minutes.

Serves 7 preschool or 5 school-age children

1 meat

❏ ❏ ❏

Green Eggs and Ham

8 eggs
1/2 cup minced fresh parsley
  (chives are also nice, but optional)
1/2 cup milk

oil
4 oz. cooked turkey ham or
  Canadian bacon
salt and pepper to taste

1. Beat eggs, parsley, and milk together.
2. Scramble egg mixture in a heavy or nonstick pan in a small amount of oil.
3. Serve with small amounts of turkey ham or Canadian bacon on the side.

Serves 8 preschool or school-age children

1 meat

Sweet Potato Fries

2 lbs. sweet potatoes or yams
1–2 t. vegetable oil

1. Peel sweet potatoes or yams and cut into sticks or wedges.
2. Toss with oil in a bowl.
3. Spread out on baking sheet.
4. Bake about 1/2 hour at 375°, or until browned and tender.
5. Sprinkle with a little salt and lemon juice, if desired.

16 vegetable servings

❏ ❏ ❏

Homemade Potato Chips
"Tato Pips"

1 lb. russet potatoes
vegetable oil

1. Preheat oven to 400°.
2. Slice potatoes paper-thin. (A food processor will make this easier.)
3. Spread the slices out in a single layer on a foil-lined or lightly oiled cookie sheet.
4. Bake for 15 or 20 minutes.
5. Remove when cooked to a crisp, golden brown.

8 vegetable servings

❏ ❏ ❏

Oven-Fried Potato Sticks
"Fiddlesticks"

4 baking potatoes, scrubbed and dried (about 2 lbs.)
1 T. oil
1/4 t. paprika

1. Cut each potato into 8–12 wedges.
2. Toss with oil and paprika.
3. Spread in shallow pan.
4. Bake until tender, 20–30 minutes at 450° or 35–40 minutes at 400°.

16 vegetable servings

Mashed Potatoes and Carrots
"Monster Mash"

1 lb. raw potatoes (russet)
1 lb. raw carrots
2 t. butter or olive oil

salt and pepper to taste
1/2 t. soy sauce (optional)

1. Wash potatoes and cut into eighths.
2. Scrub carrots and cut into 1" chunks.
3. Cook potatoes and carrots gently in about 1 cup water. If they get too dry, add a little more water. If it looks too runny, let some of the water evaporate.
4. Mash, or put in food processor, with butter, salt and pepper and the soy sauce (if desired).

Note: Thanks to Barbara Zeavin for this recipe.

16 vegetable servings

❑ ❑ ❑

Senegalese Veggie Stew

1 onion, chopped
1 T. oil
2 cups winter squash or sweet potato, peeled and cut into chunks
2 medium potatoes, cut into chunks
1 large carrot, cut into chunks
1 small bunch of greens (collards or turnip greens) or 1 10-oz. pkg. frozen greens

1/4 t. cayenne
1 cup tomato sauce
1 to 1 1/2 cups water
3/8 cup peanut butter (6 T.)
salt to taste

1. Sauté onion in oil for a few minutes.
2. Add remaining vegetables one at a time, sautéeing each for a few moments before adding the next.
3. Add cayenne, tomato sauce, and water.
4. Simmer until vegetables are tender.
5. Mix some of the broth with the peanut butter.
6. Add to the vegetables and cook another 10 minutes.
7. Taste for seasoning and add salt if desired.
8. Serve over rice or millet.

16 vegetable servings

Winter Salad

1/2 head butter lettuce
1 large carrot, grated
2 medium-sized raw beets, grated
1 package radish sprouts or 1 piece of daikon (white)
  radish about the same size as the carrot, grated*
seasoned rice vinegar to taste (the seasoned vinegar
  has some sugar and salt in it which is important
  for the flavor of this salad)

1. Arrange lettuce leaves on a platter.
2. Arrange carrot, radish sprouts or radish, and beets in separate piles on top of the lettuce. It's fun to play around with decorative patterns.
3. Sprinkle some of the vinegar over each salad before eating.

8 vegetable servings

❏ ❏ ❏

Far East Slaw

6 cups finely shredded cabbage (1 1/2 lb.)
1 red or green pepper, chopped fine
8 oz. can sliced water chestnuts
1/4 c. chopped peanuts
seasoned rice vinegar or Buttermilk Dressing to taste

1. Combine ingredients in a large bowl.
2. Dress with seasoned rice vinegar or Buttermilk Dressing (page 111).

24 vegetable servings

*Alfalfa sprouts can be substituted for radish or radish sprouts.

Shred-That-Salad!
"Confetti"

Salad Mix:
3/4 lb. green cabbage

1/2 lb. red cabbage

2 carrots

2 green peppers

1. Shred in food processor and place in large bowl.
2. Toss with either Oil and Vinegar or Curry-Yogurt Dressing.

Oil and Vinegar Dressing:
3 T. Olive oil, 3 T. vinegar, salt and pepper.

Curry-Yogurt Dressing:
6 T. yogurt, 6 T. reduced-calorie mayonnaise, 2 t. curry powder, salt.

20 vegetable servings

❏ ❏ ❏

A Different Potato Salad

4 medium potatoes, scrubbed

1 10-oz. pkg. peas and carrots

1/2 large dill pickle, chopped

1/4 cup chopped onion

2 T. plain lowfat or nonfat yogurt

2 T. reduced-fat mayonnaise

2 T. lime juice

1 t. olive oil

salt and pepper to taste

1. Steam the potatoes until tender. When cool enough to handle, cut them into cubes.
2. Steam the peas and carrots until cooked. Then cool.
3. Mix remaining ingredients in a large bowl.
4. Add the cooled potatoes, peas and carrots.
5. Chill and serve.

12 vegetable servings

Corn Soup
"Uni-corn Soup"

1 medium onion, chopped
2 t. oil
2 10-oz. pkg. frozen corn or
   fresh corn cut from 6 ears
2 1/4 cups chicken or
   vegetable broth or water

2 cups milk
1 red pepper, chopped (optional)
3/4 t. salt
1–3 cloves garlic, chopped
1/2 t. sugar

1. Sauté onion in oil until transparent.
2. Add corn, cover and let cook 15 minutes.
3. Add broth, 1 cup milk, salt, garlic and sugar.
4. Simmer for 15 more minutes.
5. Take out about 1 cup of the corn, add 1 cup milk to the pot.
6. Pureé in batches in blender until smooth.
7. Return to pot, add the reserved whole corn kernels and red pepper and heat gently.
8. Season to taste with pepper.

12 vegetable servings

❑ ❑ ❑

Creamy Winter Squash Soup

2 lbs. winter squash (butternut,
   acorn) peeled and cubed
1 onion, chopped
1 red pepper, diced
10-oz. frozen corn, or fresh corn
   cut from 2 ears

1 T. oil
2–3 t. mild curry powder
salt to taste

1. Lightly sauté onion and curry powder in oil.
2. Add squash and 3 cups water and simmer until squash is very tender.
3. Purée mixture in batches in blender.
4. Return to pot and add enough water or milk for desired consistency.
5. Add red pepper and corn, and cook gently until they are tender.
6. Add salt to taste.

16 vegetable servings

Harvest Squash Bake
"Harvest Moon Squash"

1 1/2 lb. winter squash (butternut,
  acorn, banana) peeled, seeded, and
  cut into chunks
1 apple, cored and cut into chunks

2 T. raisins or currants
1/2 cup orange juice
1 T. butter, cut into pieces

1. Stir all ingredients together.
2. Put into greased shallow baking dish.
3. Baked covered at 375° for about 45 minutes, stirring occasionally.

10 vegetable servings

❏ ❏ ❏

Cream of Broccoli Soup
"Swamp Soup"

1 1/2 lb. broccoli, chopped (include
  most of the stems)
1/2 medium onion, chopped
1 T. oil
1 potato, scrubbed and cut into chunks
1 rib celery, sliced
1 carrot, chopped

2 cups water
2 cups milk
1/2 t. nutmeg
3/4 t. salt
1/2 t. pepper (preferably fresh
  ground)

1. Sauté onion in oil.
2. Add carrot and celery and sauté for 2–3 minutes.
3. Add broccoli, potato, and water and simmer until the vegetables are quite tender.
4. Stir in 1 cup of the milk, and purée the mixture in blender or food processor.
5. Return to pan and add the other cup of milk and seasonings.
6. If too liquid, thicken with 1 T. cornstarch mixed into 2 T. cold milk and heat.

Note: Nice with parmesan cheese on top!

12 vegetable servings

Wiggly Fruit

2 t. (1 envelope) unflavored gelatin
2 cups unsweetened fruit juice (not fresh pineapple)
2–3 cups sliced fruit

1. Mix gelatin with 1/4 cup juice in a bowl.
2. Measure another 1/2 cup juice and bring to a boil.
3. Add hot juice to gelatin mixture, stirring until all of the gelatin is dissolved.
4. Add remaining juice and chill until it begins to set.
5. Add fruit, stir, and chill until firm.

Note: Strong-flavored juices like grape, cherry or raspberry work best. Apple-raspberry juice with peach slices is great!

8 fruit servings

❏ ❏ ❏

Micro-Fruit

1 lb. apples, halved and cored
or
1 lb. pears, halved and cored
or
1 lb. bananas, halved lengthwise
cinnamon, ginger, or cinnamon-sugar

1. Sprinkle fruit with cinnamon, ginger or cinnamon-sugar.
2. Place on microwave-safe dish.
3. Bake in microwave oven: pears—about 1 1/2 minutes
apples—about 3 minutes
bananas—about 45 seconds to 1 minute.

Note: This is even yummier with a spoonful of plain yogurt on top!

6 fruit servings

Soft-Serve Fruit
"Frosty Fruit"

2 lbs. bananas, peeled and cut into chunks
or
2 lbs. mangoes, peeled and cut into chunks

1. Freeze fruit (but not rock hard).
2. Run frozen fruit through food processor. (You may need to soften it up a bit first. Let it run long enough to whip a lot of air into the mixture, but not long enough to completely thaw the fruit.)
3. Serve right away.

Note: Cantaloupe, peaches or strawberries may also be used, but you will need to use a little fruit juice to get the right consistency.

12 fruit servings

❑ ❑ ❑

Pumpkin "Custard"
"Jack O'Lantern Pudding"
(no milk, no eggs)

1 15-oz. can pumpkin pureé (2 cups)   *1 t. cinnamon*
8 oz. tofu (regular or firm)   *1/4 t. ginger*
6 T. brown sugar   *1/4 t. cloves*
1 T. molasses

1. Blend all ingredients in food processor until very smooth.
2. Pour into oiled casserole.
3. Bake at 350° for 35–40 minutes.
4. Chill and serve.

Note: This can also be used as a dairyless pie filling.

7 vegetable servings

Pancake Mixtures
"Flying Saucers"

The following dry mixtures can be prepared in advance. When you wish to make pancakes, mix wet ingredients together and combine with dry mixture of your choice and cook pancakes on a lightly greased griddle.

Basic:

4 cups unbleached flour
4 cups whole wheat flour
2 cups buttermilk powder
1/4 cup sugar

4 t. baking powder
4 t. baking soda
2 t. salt

1. Combine 1 1/4 cups of dry mixture with 1 cup water, 1 egg, and 2 T. oil.

Multigrain:

1 cup unbleached flour
1 cup whole wheat flour
1 cup cornmeal
1 cup oat bran
1 cup buttermilk powder

2 T. sugar
2 t. baking powder
2 t. baking soda
1 t. salt

1. Combine 1 1/2 cups of dry mixture with 1 cup water, 1 egg and 2 T. oil.

Wheatless:

1 cup rice flour
1 cup oat bran
1 T. sugar

1 1/2 t. baking powder
1 t. soda
3/4 t. salt

1. Combine 1 cup dry mixture with 1 cup of buttermilk, 1 egg (or egg substitute) and 2 T. oil.

Eggless: Replace egg with egg substitute.

Each batch makes about 12 3-inch pancakes

Chris' Pancakes

1 cup whole wheat flour
1 cup unbleached flour
1 T. sugar
1 t. baking soda
1 t. baking powder
1/2 t. salt
1 t. cinnamon

1 t. nutmeg
1 1/2 cup buttermilk
1/2 cup orange juice
2 eggs
2 T. oil
1 t. vanilla

1. Mix dry ingredients together.
2. Mix wet ingredients together.
3. Mix wet and dry ingredients together.
4. Cook on lightly greased griddle.

Makes about 24 3" pancakes

❏ ❏ ❏

Gingerbread Pancakes
"Gingerbread Frisbees"

1 cup whole wheat flour
1 cup white flour
1/2 t. salt
1 t. soda
1 1/2–2 cups buttermilk
2 eggs

3 T. molasses
1 t. ginger
1/2 t. cinnamon
1/2 t. ground cloves
1 T. oil

1. Mix dry ingredients together.
2. Mix wet ingredients together.
3. Mix wet and dry ingredients together.
4. Cook on lightly greased griddle.

Makes about 24 3" pancakes

Banana Bread
"Banana Gorilla Bread"

1 cup regular tofu, mashed
1/3 cup oil
1 1/4 cups sugar
2 eggs, slightly beaten
2 t. vanilla
2 cups very ripe mashed bananas
   (4 large or 5 small bananas)
2 T. lemon juice

3 1/2 cups flour (can use 1 1/2 cups
   whole wheat)
2 t. soda
1 t. baking powder
1 t. salt
1 cup chopped walnuts or pecans
   (optional)

1. Blend tofu and oil in food processor or blender until very smooth.
2. Add sugar, egg, and vanilla and blend very well.
3. Add bananas and lemon juice and process briefly.
4. Combine flour, soda, baking powder and salt.
5. Gently combine the liquid and dry ingredients.
6. Fold in nuts (optional).
7. Put batter into 2 greased loaf pans.
8. Bake at 350° for 50–60 minutes or until done.

Each loaf serves 32 preschoolers or 16 school-age children
1 bread/grain

❏ ❏ ❏

Pumpkin Bread

1 cup regular tofu, mashed
1/4 cup oil
1 1/2 cup brown sugar
4 eggs
2/3 cup orange juice
1 15 1/2-oz. can pumpkin (2 cups)

3 1/2 cups flour
1 t. baking powder
2 t. baking soda
1 t. salt
2 t. cinnamon
2. t. ground cloves
1 cup currants or raisins

1. Blend oil and tofu in blender or food processor until very smooth.
2. Add sugar, eggs, orange juice, and pumpkin, and blend again.
3. Stir together dry ingredients.
4. Add to pumpkin mixture.
5. Stir in currants or raisins.
6. Pour into 2 greased loaf pans.
7. Bake at 350° for about 1 hour or until toothpick comes out clean.

Each loaf serves 32 preschoolers or 16 school-age children
1 bread/grain

Tropical Bread

1 cup whole wheat flour
2 1/2 cups unbleached flour
2 t. baking soda
1/2 t. salt
1 cup sugar

1/2 cup oil
2 eggs
2 very ripe bananas, mashed
1 cup crushed pineapple, drained
   (1 8-oz. can)
2 t. vanilla

1. Combine flours, salt and soda.
2. Cream together sugar, oil, and egg.
3. Stir in bananas and pineapple.
4. Add flour mixture, stirring gently.
5. Stir in vanilla.
6. Bake in 2 greased loaf pans at 350° for 45 minutes.

Each loaf serves 24 preschoolers or 12 school-age children
1 bread/grain

❏ ❏ ❏

"Bikini Bread"

1 cup whole wheat flour
1 cup unbleached flour
1 1/2 t. baking powder
1 t. cinnamon
1 t. ground cloves
1/4 t. baking soda
1/2 cup chopped walnuts

1/2 t. salt
1/3 cup oil
1/2 cup sugar
2 eggs
1 t. vanilla
2 cups grated zucchini

1. Sift or stir dry ingredients together.
2. Beat oil, sugar, eggs and vanilla until fluffy.
3. Add dry ingredients to wet mixture.
4. Fold in zucchini and nuts.
5. Bake in greased loaf pan at 350° for 45 minutes.

Serves 32 preschoolers or 16 school-age children
1 bread/grain

Lemon Blueberry Muffins

2 eggs
1/2 cup sugar
1/4 cup oil
7/8 cup milk
rind and juice of 1 lemon
2 cups flour (whole wheat pastry or
   1/2 whole wheat, 1/2 white)

1 T. baking powder
1/2 t. baking soda
1/2 t. salt
1 1/2 cups blueberries (dredged in
   1 T. flour)

1. Mix eggs, sugar and oil and beat until foamy.
2. Add milk and lemon.
3. Stir together flour, baking powder, soda and salt.
4. Stir into liquid ingredients until just blended.
5. Fold in blueberries gently.
6. Spoon batter into muffin cups.
7. Bake at 425° for 20 minutes.

Makes 12 muffins
1 bread/grain

❏ ❏ ❏

Crunchy Apricot Bread

1 1/4 cup dried apricots
1 cup boiling water
1/3 cup oil
1/2 cup sugar
2 eggs

2 1/4 cups unbleached flour
1 T. baking powder
1/2 t. salt
3/4 cup Grapenuts cereal
2/3 cup milk

1. Pour boiling water over apricots. Let sit for 10 minutes. Drain.
2. Beat oil, sugar and eggs until fluffy.
3. Stir together flour, baking powder, salt and Grapenuts.
4. Add flour mixture to oil, sugar, egg mixture alternately with the milk.
5. Fold in the apricots.
6. Bake in greased loaf pan at 350° for 1 hour.

Note: This can also be made with dried peaches which are cheaper and less tart.

Each loaf serves 32 preschoolers or 16 school-age children
1 bread/grain

Bulgur Pilaf

1/2 cup onion, chopped
1 T. oil
1 cup bulgur wheat
2 T. sesame seeds

2 cups water or stock
3/4 t. salt
2 t. parsley flakes
1 clove garlic, whole

1. Sauté onion in oil for 5 minutes.
2. Add bulgur and sesame seeds. Sauté for 2 minutes.
3. Add all remaining ingredients.
4. Bring to a boil, then simmer for about 15 minutes or until liquid is absorbed.
5. Remove garlic clove before serving.

Serves 12 preschool or 6 school-age children
1 bread/grain

❑   ❑   ❑

Swiss Breakfast

1 1/4 cup raw oats
1 cup water
2 T. wheat germ
2 T. honey or brown sugar

3–4 cups fresh fruit (banana,
   peaches, blueberries, grated
   apple, etc.)
1 cup plain yogurt
1 T. orange juice

1. Stir oats and water together.
2. Let sit overnight in refrigerator.
3. In the morning, stir all ingredients together and serve.

Note: Chopped toasted almonds and/or hazelnuts may be added.

Serves 8 preschool or 4 school-age children
1 bread/grain + 1 fruit

Cereal Hash

equal amounts of a variety of low-sugar cereals,
which can include naturally multi-colored cereal
rounds (available at health-food stores)

1. Mix up a variety of cereals and store in an airtight container. Aim for an interesting mix of shapes and sizes.

preschool: 1/3 cup = 1 bread/grain

school-age: 3/4 cup = 1 bread/grain

❏ ❏ ❏

Assorted Chips for Dips
"The Big Dippers"

Won Ton Chips

1 lb. wonton wrappers

1. Cut Won Ton Wrappers into triangles.
2. Place in a single layer on lightly oiled baking sheet.
3. Bake for 4–7 minutes at 400°, until lightly browned and crisp.

Serves 32 preschool or 16 school-age children

❏ ❏ ❏

Pita Points

1 lb. pita bread

1. Cut pita breads in half and separate pieces where joined at the edges.
2. Stack and cut pieces into wedges.
3. Place in a single layer on a lightly oiled baking sheet.
4. Bake 6–10 minutes at 400°, until brown and crisp.

Serves 32 preschool or 16 school-age children

Nori-Maki Rolls

You may think kids won't like sushi, but you might be surprised!

2 cups medium-grain white rice
2 1/2 cups water
3 T. rice vinegar (not the
  seasoned variety)

2 t. sugar
1 t. salt
5–6 sheets toasted seaweed
  (sushi nori)

Fillings: About 2 cups altogether (Use your imagination! This is a good way to use up little bits of leftovers):

carrots, cut into thin strips and
  steamed lightly
cucumber, cut into thin strips
spinach or chard, steamed and
  sprinkled with toasted sesame seeds
  and a little soy sauce

green onions, cut into thin strips
avocado
cooked shrimp or crab
canned or smoked salmon (lox)

1. Rinse the rice and let it drain.
2. Place rice in saucepan with water. Bring to a boil, cover, turn heat way down and cook for 20 minutes.
3. At the end of the cooking time, let the rice sit for 10–15 minutes. Resist the urge to remove the lid from the pot!
4. Turn rice out into a large bowl or roasting pan. Sprinkle the vinegar, salt, and sugar over it and mix well.
5. Allow rice to cool to room temperature.
6. Place a sheet of the seaweed (shiny side down) on a cutting board. The short side should be top-to-bottom.
7. Wet your hands and spread with 3/4–1 cup of the rice, leaving about 1/2 inch border at the bottom and 1 inch at the top.
8. Make an indentation in the rice horizontally along the middle. Arrange your choice of fillings over this. (It's OK if it's humped up).
9. Start rolling from the bottom, squeezing with both hands as you go. Moisten the top border of the seaweed with some water and keep rolling until the end.
10. Cover rolls tightly with plastic wrap and refrigerate until ready to serve (up to 48 hours, depending on the fillings).
11. At serving time, cut each roll with a sharp knife into 8 pieces and arrange on a platter. Mustard and pickled ginger are good accompaniments.

Serves 20 preschool or 10 school-age children
1 bread/grain

Mock Sour Cream
"Make Believe Sour Cream"

2 cups cottage cheese
2 T. lemon juice
2 T. lowfat milk

1. Run ingredients through food processor or blender until absolutely silky smooth. Makes about 2 cups.

❑ ❑ ❑

Creamy Dill Dip
"Dippity Doo Dah Dip"

2 t. parsley flakes
2 small garlic cloves, pressed
1 t. dill weed

1. Add to 2 cups Mock Sour Cream.

Serves 16 preschool or 8 school-age children for snack.
1 meat alternative

❑ ❑ ❑

Toasted Onion Dip

2 T. dry minced onion, toasted lightly
    3–5 minutes at 350°
2 t. soy sauce
dash of garlic powder

1. Add to 2 cups Mock Sour Cream.

Serves 16 preschool or 8 school-age children for snack.
1 meat alternative

Buttermilk Dressing
"Brontosaurus Milk Dressing"

1 cup buttermilk
1/2 cup mayonnaise
1/2 t. pepper
2 t. dried minced onion

1/2 t. garlic powder
1/4 t. salt
1 t. parsley flakes
1/4 t. dill weed

1. Whisk ingredients together.
2. Let sit for at least 1 hour to blend flavors before using.

❏   ❏   ❏

Bean Dip
"Mud Dip"

1 1/2 cups cooked (or canned) pinto beans
1 T. Mexican spice mix (below)
6 oz. grated jack or Cheddar cheese

1. Mash beans with a fork or potato masher.
2. Stir in spice mix and grated cheese.
3. Heat until cheese melts, on the stove or in microwave.

Mexican Spice Mix: 1/4 t. garlic powder
1 T. onion powder
1 T. cumin
2 T. chili powder

Serves 24 preschool or 12 school-age children for snack
1 meat alternative

❏   ❏   ❏

Hummous
"Quicksand"

2 cups chickpeas (16-oz. can)
1 T. tahini
1 T. lemon juice
1 clove garlic, pressed
1/2 t. cumin

1/4 t. paprika
1/4 t. salt
1 t. olive oil
1/4 cup water

1. Blend all ingredients except water in food processor.
2. Add water 1 T. at a time, until you have the right consistency (a fairly thick purée).
3. Process until very smooth.
4. Use as spread with crackers or pita bread.

Serves 12 preschool or 6 school-age children for snack
1 meat alternative

❑ ❑ ❑

Savory Scrambled Cereals

5 cups unsweetened or low-sugar
   cereals, mixed (e.g., Cheerios,
   Wheat Chex, Rice Chex, Corn Chex,
   Crispix, Kix, Shredded Wheat)
1 cup small pretzel rings*
1 cup unsalted, roasted peanuts*

2 T. margarine
1 T. Worchestershire sauce
1 t. Spike seasoning
1/8 t. garlic powder

1. Melt margarine in a roasting pan in 250° oven.
2. Stir Worchestershire and seasonings into the melted margarine.
3. Toss in cereals and pretzels and peanuts (optional), stirring gently to coat.
4. Bake at 250° for 30–45 minutes, stirring about every 15 minutes, until toasty.

Serves (approximately) 15 preschool or 7 school-age children
1 bread/grain

*Omit for children under 5 years old.

Rice Cake Snacks
"Saucy Cheese Cake"

1 rice cake
2 T. grated Cheddar or jack cheese
salsa

1. Spread cheese on rice cake.
2. Bake at 350° until cheese melts.
3. Top with salsa.

1 per preschool or 2 per school-age child for snack
1 bread + 1 meat alternative

❑ ❑ ❑

"Pizza Cake"

1 rice cake
2 T. "instant" pizza sauce (page 115)
2 T. grated mozzarella cheese

1. Spread sauce, then cheese on rice cake.
2. Bake at 350° until cheese melts.

Note: Can be microwaved, but they get soft.

1 per preschool or 2 per school-age child for snack
1 bread + 1 meat alternative

Peanut Butter Ping Pong Balls

Version I:

1/2 cup peanut butter
1/4 cup honey

1/2 t. vanilla
2–3 cups Rice Krispies or
    crispy brown rice cereal

1. Stir together peanut butter, honey and vanilla.
2. Stir in cereal.
3. Wet hands and form the mixture into balls.
4. Place on waxed paper and chill. Store in covered container in refrigerator.

Version II:

1/2 cup peanut butter
1/4 cup molasses

1/2 t. cinnamon
2–3 cups Rice Krispies or
    crispy brown rice cereal

Repeat directions as above.

Serves 6 preschool or 4 school-age children for snack
1 meat alternative + 1 bread/grain

❑ ❑ ❑

Build-a-Sundae

1 1/2 cups yogurt or cottage cheese
1 lb. chopped fruits
optional toppings:
  • nuts
  • unsweetened cereals
  • honey or maple syrup (optional)

1. Put yogurt or cottage cheese in individual bowls.
2. Add fruits (applesauce, raisins, chopped dates, berries, bananas, etc.).
3. Top with nuts, cereals, and/or honey or maple syrup (optional).

Serves 6 preschoolers or 3 school-age children for snack
1 meat alternative + 1 fruit

"Instant" Pizza Sauce

2 cups canned crushed tomatoes *1 1/2 t. oregano*
3/4 t. garlic powder *1/2 t. salt*
1 t. basil *1/4 t. pepper*

1. Stir all ingredients together.
2. Let sit at least 1 hour.
3. Use as sauce for pizzas.

Makes 2 cups

❑ ❑ ❑

Quick Pizzas
"Road Runner Pizza"

For each child:

*Base: English muffin half, or flour tortilla, or pita bread,
split, or slice of french bread*

2 T. Instant Pizza Sauce (recipe above)
*2–4 T. (1/2–1 oz.) cheese—mozzarella, Cheddar,
jack, provolone, or a mixture, grated or sliced*

1. Spread Instant Pizza Sauce over base.
2. Cover with cheese and any other toppings you fancy.
3. Bake at 425° until bubbly.

Toppings: sliced mushrooms, green peppers, onions, olives, artichoke hearts . . .

1 meat alternative + 1 bread per serving for snack

❑ ❑ ❑

Sunshine Dip

2 cups plain nonfat or lowfat yogurt
2 T. orange juice concentrate

1. Mix together.
2. You can experiment with concentrates of other juices, too! Try grapefruit, tangerine, lemonade, or limeade.
3. Use as a dip for pieces of raw fruit—peaches, strawberries, kiwi, bananas . . .

Serves 8 preschoolers or 4 school-age children for snack
1 meat alternative

Frosty Fruit Shakes

Peanut Butter Banana

2 cups milk or 1 1/2 cups plain yogurt
2-3 bananas, frozen (about 1 lb.)
3 T. peanut butter

Liquid Sunshine

2 cups milk or 1 1/2 cups plain yogurt
1 cup crushed pineapple
2–3 bananas, frozen (about 1 lb.)
1/2 t. vanilla

Bananaberry

2 cups milk or 1 1/2 cups plain yogurt
2–3 bananas, frozen (about 1 lb.)
1 cup strawberries or blueberries (may be frozen)
1/2 t. vanilla

Spicy Apple

1 1/2 cups plain yogurt
2 cups chunky applesauce
1/2 t. cinnamon
(ice cubes or crushed ice)

Each recipe serves 4 preschool or 2 school-age children
1 milk (or 1 meat alternative if yogurt is used) + 1 fruit

❑ ❑ ❑

Hot Chocolate

4 cups milk
1 1/2 T cocoa powder
1 1/2 T sugar

1. Combine cocoa powder and sugar with about 1/4 cup of milk.
2. Whisk in the remaining milk.
3. Cook over medium heat, stirring constantly, until milk is hot but not boiling. Or heat in microwave 2–3 minutes, or until milk is hot.

Serves 8 preschool or 4 school-age children
1 milk

CHAPTER FIVE

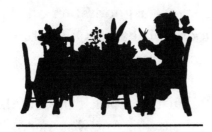

Sample Menus
Using Our Recipes

Ten Breezy Breakfasts

It's easy to help children get a good start on the day when you have healthful make-ahead foods on hand. Quick breads and muffins can be made in large batches and frozen until needed. The dry ingredients for pancakes can be measured out the night before or made up in large quantities as a "mix." You can cook hot cereals and stew fruit very successfully in a microwave oven. And you needn't restrict your thinking to traditional "breakfast foods." Sandwiches and even pasta can taste great in the morning!

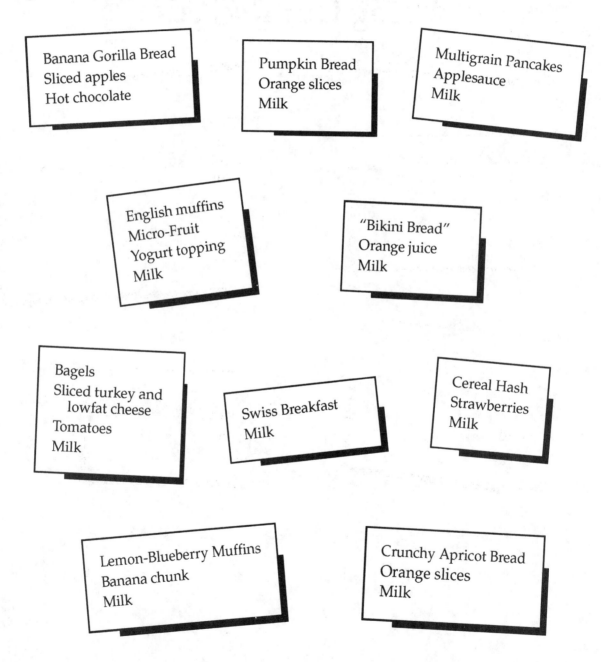

Banana Gorilla Bread
Sliced apples
Hot chocolate

Pumpkin Bread
Orange slices
Milk

Multigrain Pancakes
Applesauce
Milk

English muffins
Micro-Fruit
Yogurt topping
Milk

"Bikini Bread"
Orange juice
Milk

Bagels
Sliced turkey and
    lowfat cheese
Tomatoes
Milk

Swiss Breakfast
Milk

Cereal Hash
Strawberries
Milk

Lemon-Blueberry Muffins
Banana chunk
Milk

Crunchy Apricot Bread
Orange slices
Milk

Fine Finger Feasts

Most children love eating with their hands. While we certainly think that they should get lots of practice with flatware, we know that meals that can be eaten entirely with the fingers are a fun change of pace. They're also easy on the cook.

Chicken Fingers
Bread sticks
Assorted raw vegetables
Apple wedges
Milk

Cold sliced omelets
Nori-Maki rolls
Sliced cucumbers
Tangerines
Milk

(Cold) Turkey Loaf cubes
Oven-Fried Potato Sticks
Broccoli and carrot sticks
Crackers
Milk

Bean Dip
Tortillas (corn or flour), heated and cut into strips or wedges
Cherry tomatoes
Lettuce
Fresh pineapple spears
Milk

Homemade Fish Sticks
Sweet Potato Fries
Zucchini and green pepper strips
Bread
Milk

Quick Pizzas
Assorted raw vegetables
Apples
Milk

Teddy Bear Tea Parties

Tea parties, complete with teddy bears or other favorite stuffed animals, are a delightful and relaxing ritual for snacktime. The "tea" can actually be warmed apple cider, hot cocoa, or basic herbal tea, such as peppermint (chamomile, while mild, can cause problems for children with ragweed allergies). If you have some sturdy teacups by all means use them. Lots of foods are appropriate for teatime . . . as long as they are dainty.

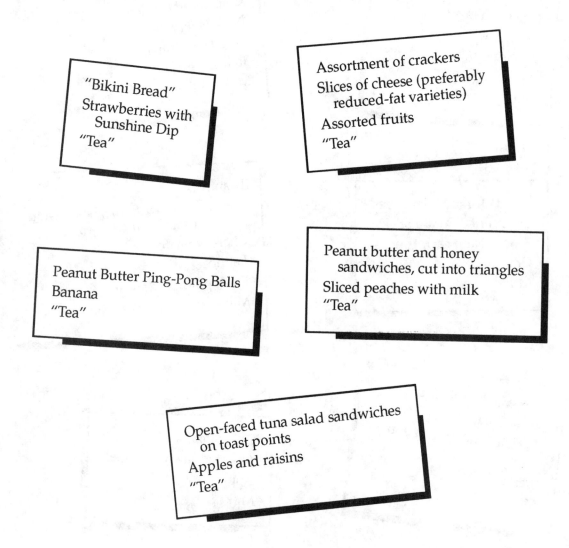

"Bikini Bread"
Strawberries with
Sunshine Dip
"Tea"

Assortment of crackers
Slices of cheese (preferably
reduced-fat varieties)
Assorted fruits
"Tea"

Peanut Butter Ping-Pong Balls
Banana
"Tea"

Peanut butter and honey
sandwiches, cut into triangles
Sliced peaches with milk
"Tea"

Open-faced tuna salad sandwiches
on toast points
Apples and raisins
"Tea"

Lunch Around the World

Few of the ethnic recipes in this book are authentic. That's because we found that traditional preparation methods were too lengthy, ingredients were difficult to find, or the authentic versions contained too much fat or salt. Similarly, the menus listed below are not truly representative of meals eaten in certain cultures. However, these menus do illustrate typical flavor principles of a variety of cuisines and include foods that might be eaten together in a meal. If you're interested in presenting truly ethnic meals to the children, ask friends or the children's parents for family recipes and menu outlines.

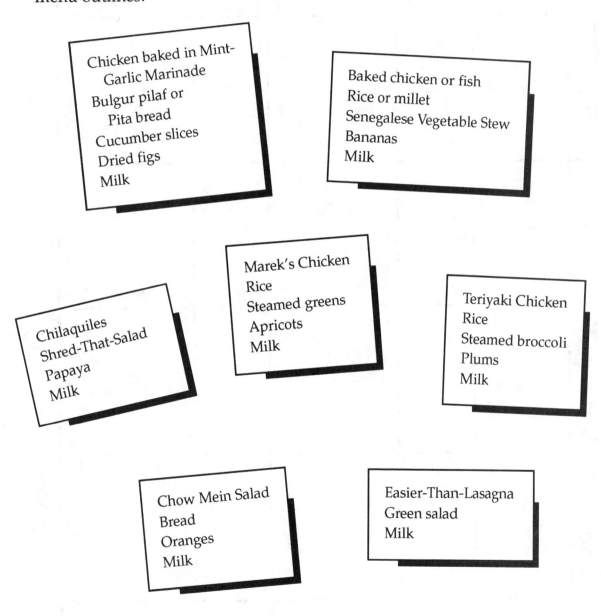

Chicken baked in Mint-
Garlic Marinade
Bulgur pilaf or
Pita bread
Cucumber slices
Dried figs
Milk

Baked chicken or fish
Rice or millet
Senegalese Vegetable Stew
Bananas
Milk

Chilaquiles
Shred-That-Salad
Papaya
Milk

Marek's Chicken
Rice
Steamed greens
Apricots
Milk

Teriyaki Chicken
Rice
Steamed broccoli
Plums
Milk

Chow Mein Salad
Bread
Oranges
Milk

Easier-Than-Lasagna
Green salad
Milk

Meal Planner

Week of: _____

Meals	Monday	Tuesday	Wednesday	Thursday	Friday
Breakfast Bread or Grain Fruit or Veggie Milk					
Snack Choose from 2 groups					
Lunch Bread or Grain "Meat" Vegetable Fruit or Veggie Milk					
Snack Choose from 2 groups					
Supper Bread or Grain "Meat" Vegetable Fruit or Veggie Milk					

✐✓ *Shopping List*

☐ **Fresh Fruits**
- ☐ _____ ☐ _____
- ☐ _____ ☐ _____
- ☐ _____ ☐ _____
- ☐ _____ ☐ _____
- ☐ _____ ☐ _____

☐ **Fresh Vegetables**
- ☐ _____ ☐ _____
- ☐ _____ ☐ _____
- ☐ _____ ☐ _____
- ☐ _____ ☐ _____
- ☐ _____ ☐ _____

☐ **Frozen Foods**
- ☐ _____ ☐ _____
- ☐ _____ ☐ _____
- ☐ _____ ☐ _____
- ☐ _____ ☐ _____
- ☐ _____ ☐ _____

☐ **Poultry/Fish/Meat**
- ☐ _____ ☐ _____
- ☐ _____ ☐ _____
- ☐ _____ ☐ _____
- ☐ _____ ☐ _____

☐ **Dairy Products**
- ☐ _____ ☐ _____
- ☐ _____ ☐ _____
- ☐ _____ ☐ _____
- ☐ _____ ☐ _____

☐ **Staples**
- ☐ _____ ☐ _____
- ☐ _____ ☐ _____
- ☐ _____ ☐ _____
- ☐ _____ ☐ _____
- ☐ _____ ☐ _____

☐ **Breads/Cereals/Grains**
- ☐ _____ ☐ _____
- ☐ _____ ☐ _____
- ☐ _____ ☐ _____
- ☐ _____ ☐ _____
- ☐ _____ ☐ _____
- ☐ _____ ☐ _____
- ☐ _____

☐ **Canned Goods**
- ☐ _____ ☐ _____
- ☐ _____ ☐ _____
- ☐ _____ ☐ _____
- ☐ _____ ☐ _____
- ☐ _____ ☐ _____
- ☐ _____

☐ **Baking Supplies**
- ☐ _____ ☐ _____
- ☐ _____ ☐ _____
- ☐ _____ ☐ _____
- ☐ _____ ☐ _____

☐ **Beverages**
- ☐ _____ ☐ _____
- ☐ _____ ☐ _____
- ☐ _____ ☐ _____

☐ **Spices/Condiments**
- ☐ _____ ☐ _____
- ☐ _____ ☐ _____
- ☐ _____ ☐ _____
- ☐ _____ ☐ _____

☐ **Other Items**
- ☐ _____ ☐ _____
- ☐ _____ ☐ _____
- ☐ _____ ☐ _____
- ☐ _____ ☐ _____
- ☐ _____ ☐ _____
- ☐ _____ ☐ _____

☐ **Paper Products**
- ☐ _____ ☐ _____
- ☐ _____ ☐ _____
- ☐ _____ ☐ _____

☐ **Cleaning Supplies**
- ☐ _____ ☐ _____
- ☐ _____ ☐ _____
- ☐ _____ ☐ _____

☐ **Household Items**
- ☐ _____ ☐ _____
- ☐ _____ ☐ _____
- ☐ _____ ☐ _____
- ☐ _____ ☐ _____
- ☐ _____ ☐ _____
- ☐ _____ ☐ _____

CHAPTER SIX

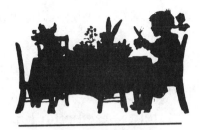

Running a Ship-Shape Kitchen

How to Save Money on Food

You don't have to spend a lot of money to provide good nutrition. Some of the most nutritious foods are very inexpensive, and some expensive foods aren't very healthful. So go ahead, save some money . . . you aren't being cheap, you're being smart!

- ❏ Decide how much money you can spend on food.
- ❏ Plan menus ahead of time. Make a shopping list and stick to it!
- ❏ Shop no more than once a week. The more often you walk into a store, the more you'll be tempted by impulse items.
- ❏ Serve less meat and more beans, grains, fruits, and vegetables.
- ❏ Have children drink water instead of juice or milk when they're thirsty between meals.
- ❏ Be very careful to transport and store foods properly so they don't spoil before you can use them.
- ❏ Use leftovers, but handle them carefully!
- ❏ Have a garden and grow your own (or let the children do it).

❑ Shop smart . . .

- Eat before you go shopping.

- Leave children at home, unless you can say "no" and mean it!

- *Read labels* . . . know what you're buying.

- Compare unit ("per pound") prices to decide which size and brand of an item is the better buy. See *Anatomy of a Shelf Pricing Label* (page 127).

- Compare the price of convenience foods with their "from scratch" counterparts.

- Be aware of the high cost of packaging. Buy in bulk when you can.

- Take advantage of seasonal specials on produce, meats, and groceries.

- Buy house brands rather than name brands when their quality suits you as well.

- Don't run all over town to save ten cents; you'll spend more on gas!

- Use coupons *when they're for items you would use anyway.*

- Look into opportunities for cooperative food buying with other families, child care providers, or feeding programs.

- *Buy only what you can use.*

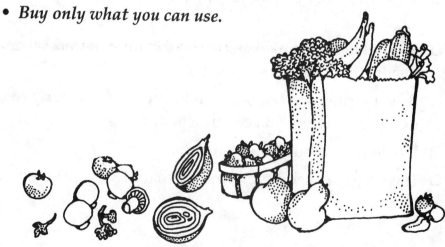

Anatomy of a Shelf Pricing Label

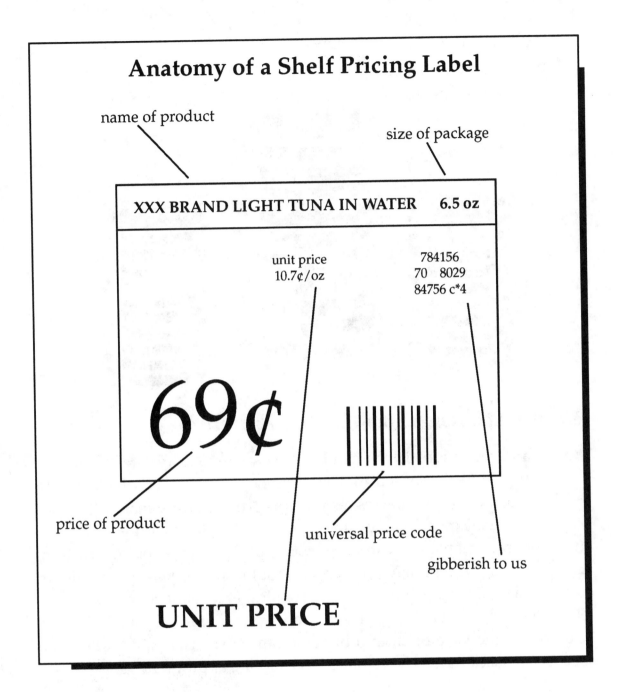

name of product

size of package

XXX BRAND LIGHT TUNA IN WATER   6.5 oz

unit price
10.7¢/oz

784156
70   8029
84756 c*4

69¢

price of product

universal price code

gibberish to us

UNIT PRICE

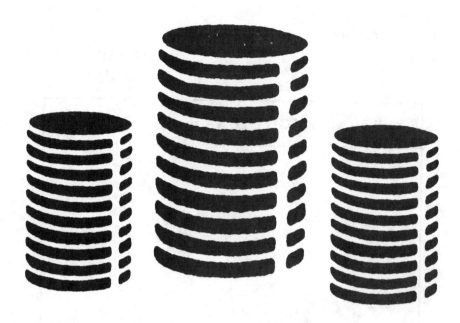

How Much Am I Spending on Protein?

Meats and meat substitutes can be the most expensive items on your menu. If you are interested in saving money on food, you have several options. You can serve the less expensive protein foods more often. You can combine inexpensive and more costly protein foods at the same meal (for example, bean chili with cheese on top). You can avoid overloading children with high-protein foods (you should offer at least the minimum serving size, of course, but you really shouldn't feel obliged to offer a child 9 ounces of chicken at one sitting). And if you would like your children to experience the taste of shrimp or some other expensive food, you could serve it at snack time, when smaller servings are appropriate.

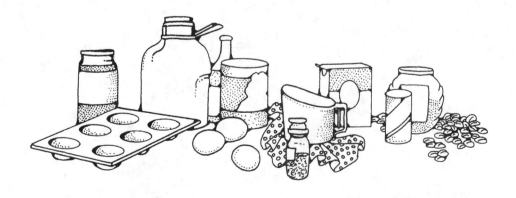

We walked through our local supermarket and took note of the prices currently charged for various meats and meat substitutes. Then we calculated what it would cost to provide a lunchtime serving to a preschooler. Some of our results surprised us!

Food Item	Cost per serving (1–1/2 oz/equiv)*
Lentils, dried	$ .03
Pinto beans, dried	.05
Eggs	.09
Canned chickpeas	.17
Turkey franks	.18
Canned tuna, water pack	.20
Cottage cheese	.26
Lean ground beef	.26
Chicken drumsticks	.27
Peanut butter, natural	.29
Cheddar cheese, store brand	.34
Frozen fish sticks	.38
Ground turkey	.38
Chicken breasts (bone in)	.44
Parmesan cheese, store brand	.45
Fried snapper fillets	.47
Pork chops	.81

Price isn't everything, and you should consider whether a food has much to offer nutritionally, as well. Turkey franks are relatively cheap, but they are also high in fat and sodium. Ground turkey is costlier than ground beef, but it is much lower in saturated fat.

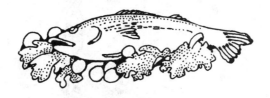

*Depending on where you get your food, of course, your actual costs will differ.

Don't Let Those Nutrients Get Away!

Nutrients can be destroyed when foods aren't handled properly. Long storage times, exposure to air and light, and prolonged cooking are notorious nutrient-robbers. Make the foods you serve as nutritious as possible by following these basic guidelines:

Buy it right

❑ Avoid food that looks wilted, bruised, or spoiled.

❑ Check expiration dates on packages.

❑ Fresh produce is generally preferable. However, fruits and vegetables that have been sitting in storage or in produce bins for a long time will gradually lose their advantage. In that case, frozen foods will be better. Some foods that don't freeze well, like tomatoes and pineapple, are OK canned.

Store it right

❑ When you're taking food home from the store, or if you've received a delivery of perishable foods, don't delay putting them away.

❑ Keep foods at the proper temperature:

65° or below for canned foods

40° or below in the refrigerator

0° or below in the freezer.

❑ Use foods within their recommended storage times (see *How Long Will It Keep?*, pags 132–133).

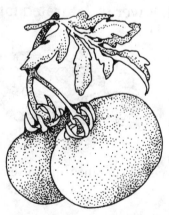

Cook it right

- ❑ Don't overcook foods.

- ❑ Serve raw fruits and vegetables often.

- ❑ Wash produce before cooking or serving, but don't soak it.

- ❑ Cut fruits and vegetables as close to serving time as possible. If you must prepare them ahead of time, seal in air-tight bags and refrigerate.

- ❑ Cook vegetables in a minimum of water and only until tender-crisp. Steaming, microwaving, and pressure-cooking are better than boiling.

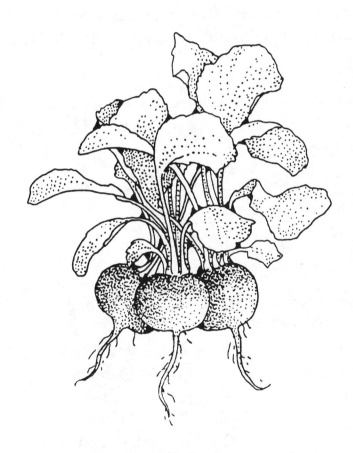

How Long Will It Keep?

	Canned/ Pantry (months)	Refrigerator (days)	Freezer (months)
Produce			
Asparagus	6	4–6	8–10
Broccoli	—	3–5	10–12
Carrots	12	7–14	10–12
Corn	12	1	10–12
Greens	12	1–2	10–12
Lettuce	—	7–10	—
Green peppers	—	4–5	10–12
Onions	1–3 weeks	—	—
Potatoes	1–2 weeks	—	—
Sweet potatoes	5–7 days	—	—
Tomatoes	6	1–2	2
Apples	12	2–4	10–12
Bananas	—	7	3
Grapefruit	6	10–14	10–12
Oranges	6	10–14	10–12
Peaches	12	3–5	10–12
Strawberries	—	3–5	10–12
Watermelon	—	7	10–12
Dairy Products			
Butter	—	1–3 months	6–9
Cheese, Cheddar	—	1–2 months	6
Cheese, cottage	—	7	—
Cheese, mozzarella	—	2–4 weeks	6
Cheese, Parmesan		12 months	—
Fluid milk	—	1–5	3
Infant formula	12–18	2 (opened)	—
Nonfat milk powder	12	2–3 months	—
Puddings, etc., with milk	—	2–3	1
Yogurt	—	7–14	1

	Canned/ Pantry (months)	Refrigerator (days)	Freezer (months)
Meats/ Meat Substitutes			
Beans, dried	12	—	—
Beef, roast	—	3–5	6–12
Beef, ground	—	1–2	2–4
Beef, cooked in casserole	—	3	2–3
Beef, cooked in gravy	—	1–2	2–3
Chicken parts	—	1	6–9
Chicken, cooked, plain	—	3–4	1
Chicken, cooked, in sauce	—	1–2	6
Eggs, fresh	—	4–5 weeks	—
Eggs, hardboiled, in shell	—	2–3 weeks	—
Eggs, hardboiled, peeled	—	7	—
Fish, fatty	—	1	3
Fish, lean	—	1	6
Frankfurters	—	4–7	2
Frozen prepared entrees	—	—	2–3
Peanut butter	12	3–4 months	—
Turkey parts	—	1–2	3–6
Grain Products			
Breads, tortillas	2–4 days	4–7	4
Cereal, cooked	—	2–3	—
Cereal, ready-to-eat			
opened	3	—	—
unopened	12	—	—
Pancakes, waffles	—	1	2–3
Oats, rolled	12	—	—
Wheat flour, unbleached	6–12	12 months	12
Whole wheat flour	1	12 months	12

Source: Bailey, Janice: *Keeping Food Fresh.* New York: Harper & Row, Publishers, 1989.

Know Your Ingredients

- *Honey, brown sugar, and turbinado ("raw") sugar* are not much more nutritious than white table sugar. In the case of honey and "raw" sugar, you pay a lot more for trace amounts of vitamins and minerals. Honey and brown sugar can lend a unique taste to a recipe, however. We urge you to exercise moderation in the use of **all** sweetners.

- *Peanut butter* often has shortening and sugar added, which contribute nothing worthwhile nutritionally. Buy "natural" peanut butter made only from peanuts. It tends to separate, so stir it up after you open the jar and refrigerate it.

- Foods labeled *"sugar free"* may contain artificial sweeteners. Check the ingredients, and if the food is artificially sweetened, avoid serving it to children. Artificial sweeteners can cause diarrhea in susceptible children.[7] They can also train children to expect a very sweet taste in foods.

- *Tofu* is sometimes called "soy cheese" or "soy bean curd." It is made from soy milk and though rather bland by itself, is much appreciated by vegetarian (and non-vegetarian) cooks for its ability to accept a wide variety of seasonings. It is a good source of protein, low in saturated fat, and can be a good source of calcium if it is made with calcium sulfate. As this book goes to press, tofu is not yet acceptable for reimbursement under child feeding program guidelines. However, we feel that since it is a healthful food that many children like, it may be worth your while to serve a little of it along with other reimbursible items. We also found that it makes a nice replacement for some of the fat in quick breads and muffins, so you will see it as an ingredient in some of our recipes.

- *Bulgur* is cracked parboiled wheat. It cooks very quickly and is terrific in pilafs and salads.

- Look for *whole-grain or enriched cornmeal,* not the degerminated variety, for baking. *Polenta,* or coarsely ground corn meal, is cooked like a hot cereal.

❑ *Whole wheat pastry flour* is best for making muffins and quick breads; regular *whole wheat flour* is used in making yeasted breads.

❑ The flavors of *fresh garlic, fresh ginger, and fresh onion* are far superior to their dehydrated and powdered versions. However, when saving time is a consideration, you may need to use the processed forms of these seasonings.

❑ We suggest that you use *reduced-sodium soy sauce* in place of regular soy sauce . . . same rich flavor, less sodium.

❑ Our preferred vegetable oils for cooking are *olive oil* and *canola oil,* both of which are low in saturated fat and high in monounsaturated fat. Both are high in fat and calories, though (about 2,000 calories per cup!), so use as little as you can to get the job done.

❑ *Toasted sesame oil,* which you may also see as "oriental sesame oil," is a very dark and richy-flavored oil that is added sparingly to some Asian dishes. Light-colored sesame oil won't do the trick.

❑ *Spike,* and its low-sodium counterpart *Vegit,* are seasoning blends available in most health food stores and some supermarkets. They happen to be our favorites, but there are other blends you can try as well: *Parsley Patch* and *Mrs. Dash* are two of them. Some low-sodium seasonings are quite peppery and may be too "hot" for children, so shop around until you find one everybody likes. We suggest that you avoid any seasoning mixtures containing monosodium glutamate (MSG).

❑ *Ground turkey* can be used in place of ground beef in most recipes, or even substituted for half the beef, and is lower in fat. You have to be careful when you cook it, as it can get dry and tough when cooked too long; cook just until no pink remains.

How to Get the Most Information From a Product Label

The nutrition label on a food product should help you decide whether it would be a good choice for a healthful diet. Unfortunately, food labels as they are now used cause a lot of confusion. As this book goes to press, new regulations are being formulated that should make food labels more helpful. In the meantime, here's some information that will help you separate fact from fantasy when you're reading the information on a box of cereal or can of juice![3]

❑ Nutrition labeling is not *required* on all packaged foods. Foods must be labeled if they have been fortified with vitamins, minerals, or protein, or if a claim is being made regarding the nutrient content of the product. Some manufacturers label their food products voluntarily.

❑ A nutrition label must list the calorie, protein, carbohydrate, fat, sodium, iron, vitamins A and C, calcium, thiamin, riboflavin, and niacin content of the product. Remember, though, that these aren't the only nutrients you need.

❑ Check the serving size carefully. Sometimes unreasonably small or large serving sizes are listed in order to make the product seem more nutritionally desirable (low in calories, for example).

❑ Most foods at least have ingredient lists on their labels. The ingredients are listed in order by weight, from the most to the least. For example, if butter is the first ingredient on the list, there is more butter in the product than any other ingredient.

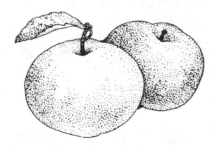

❑ You will need to know alternative names for certain food components in order to really get a clear picture of how much of them a product contains.

Sugar:	brown sugar	dextrose
	honey	fructose
	corn syrup	sucrose
	corn syrup solids	maltose
	invert sugar	molasses
	maple syrup	
Sodium:	salt	monosodium glutamate
	baking soda	sodium benzoate
	sodium caseinate	sodium nitrate
	sodium nitrite	sodium phosphate
	sodium propionate	

❑ The fat content of a food is listed in grams. But what you're probably interested in is "what's the amount of fat here relative to the calories?" There are two ways you can find this out. One is to perform some quick math: Each gram of fat has 9 calories. Multiply the grams of fat in a serving by 9 to get the calories contributed from fat. Divide this product by the total number of calories and multiply by 100. Voila! You've calculated the percentage of calories from fat. Alternatively, you can use a handy little gadget called a "Fat Finder" that does the math for you.

> **Fat Finder®**
> $5.45 from Vitaerobics
> 41-905 Boardwalk, Suite B
> Palm Desert, CA 92260-5141
> (800) 323-8042

❑ Don't be misled by percentage signs. A food that's labeled "95% fatfree" does not get just 5% of its calories from fat. It contains 5% fat by *weight*, and the heaviest component of many foods is water. Since fat has a lot of calories, the food could still be relatively high in fat.

❑ Know what the various terms on labels *really* mean:

- sodium-free = less than 5 mg sodium/serving
- very low sodium = 35 mg or less sodium/serving
- low sodium = 140 mg or less sodium/serving
- reduced sodium = at least a 75% reduction in sodium compared with the usual product
- unsalted, no salt added = no salt added during processing of a food usually made with salt
- cholesterol-free = 2 mg or less cholesterol/serving
- low cholesterol = 20 mg or less cholesterol/serving
- reduced cholesterol = 75% or more reduction in cholesterol from the usual product
- extra lean = meat or poultry contains no more than 5% fat by weight
- lean, lowfat = meat or poultry contains no more than 10% fat by weight
- light, leaner = meat or poultry that has a 25% or more reduction in fat from the usual product

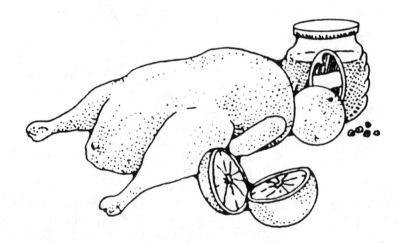

Basic Equivalents and Substitutions

Here is a listing of some common foods for which you may need to convert measurements or substitute an ingredient in a recipe. You may want to reduce the amount of fat or sugar in a recipe, or change other ingredients for health-related reasons. Or, you might discover you are out of an ingredient in the middle of preparing a meal and prefer not to dash to the store with a group of little ones in tow.

Food	Amount	Equivalent or Substitute
Apples, raw, whole	1 lb.	3 cups, pared and sliced
Apricots	1 lb. dried	5 1/2 lb. fresh
Bacon	—	For similar flavor with much less fat use Canadian bacon or boiled or baked ham
Baking powder	1 teaspoon	1/4 t. baking soda + 5/8 t. cream of tartar *or* 1/4 t. baking soda + 1/2 cup buttermilk or yogurt (reduce other liquid by 1/2 cup)
Bananas	3–4 medium	1 lb. or 1 3/4 cup mashed
Bread crumbs	1 cup	4 slices dry, 2 slices soft *or* use 3/4 cup cracker or cereal crumbs
Butter or margarine	1 cup	2 sticks
Buttermilk	1 cup	1 cup yogurt, *or* 1 cup skim or 1% milk with 2 T. vinegar or lemon juice (let stand 5 min.)
Cabbage	1 lb.	4 cups shredded
Carrots	1 lb.	3 cups shredded; 2 1/2 cups diced
Catsup or chili sauce	1 cup	1 cup tomato sauce + 1/4 cup sugar and 2 T. vinegar + spices
Cream cheese	1 cup	1 cup low fat cottage cheese with 1/4 cup margarine (lower in saturated fat and cholesterol, but not in total fat)

Food	Amount	Equivalent or Substitute
Eggs	1 cup	About 5 large eggs (in recipes using 1 or 2 eggs, 2 egg whites can be substituted for each yolk)
Yolks	1 cup	12 large yolks
Whites	1 cup	8–10 large whites
Dried	1 whole egg	2 1/2 T. beaten with 2 1/2 T. water
Flour, all purpose	1 lb.	4 cups
Flour, for thickening	1 T.	1 1/2 t. cornstarch *or* 1 T. quick cooking tapioca, *or* 2 T. granule (e.g., rice or wheat) cereal
Flour, cake	1 cup	7/8 cup sifted all-purpose flour (or, 1 cup less 2 T.)
Garlic	1 medium clove	1/8 t. garlic powder
Herbs, fresh, chopped	1 T.	1 t. dried
Lemon juice	1 t.	1/2 t. vinegar
Milk, skim	1 cup	1/3 cup instant nonfat dry milk + 7/8 cup water; for cake and muffin recipes fruit juice can be used instead of milk (for acidic juices add 1/2 t. baking soda to the recipe)
Milk, whole	1 cup	1 cup skim milk + 2 T. melted butter or margarine, *or* 1/2 cup evaporated milk + 1/2 cup water
Milk, sour	1 cup	Add 1 T. vinegar or lemon juice to 1 cup minus 1 T. milk. Let stand 5 minutes
Oranges	1 medium	5–6 T. juice; 2 to 3 T. grated rind
Rice	2 cups uncooked	6 cups cooked
Raisins, seedless	1 lb.	2 3/4 cups

Food	Amount	Equivalent or Substitute
Sour cream	1 cup	1 cup low-fat cottage cheese or part-skim ricotta puréed in blender with yogurt or buttermilk to desired consistency, *or* blend cheese with 1 T. skim milk and 1 T. lemon juice
Sugar, granulated white	1 lb.	2 1/4 cups; most standard dessert recipes can be reduced by one third to one-half the amount recommended
" " "	1 cup	3/4 cup honey + reduce liquid by 1/8 cup
" " "	"	3/4 maple syrup + reduce liquid by 1/8 cup
" " "	"	1/2 cup molasses
" " "	"	1 1/2 cup barley malt and rice syrup + reduce liquid slightly
" " "	"	1 cup date sugar
" " "	"	1 1/2 cup fruit juice concentrate + reduce liquid by 1/8 cup
" " "	"	1 cup brown sugar, packed
Tomatoes, fresh	1 lb.	1 cup tomato sauce
juice	1 cup	1/2 cup tomato sauce + 1/2 cup water
paste	1/4 cup	1/2 cup tomato sauce simmered to equal 1/4 cup paste
sauce	2 cups	3/4 cup tomato paste + 1 cup water
soup	10 3/4 oz. can	1 cup tomato sauce + 1/4 cup water
Yogurt	1 cup	1 cup buttermilk

Basic Guide to Measurements

Reminder: Help with measuring is a great way to enable children to participate in the cooking process. In fact, checking the accuracy of your measuring equipment can make an interesting math and science activity.

Standard U.S. Liquid Measurements

3 teaspoons	=	1 tablespoon
4 tablespoons	=	1/4 cup or 2 ounces
5 1/3 tablespoons	=	1/3 cup or 2 2/3 ounces
12 tablespoons	=	3/4 cup or 6 ounces
16 tablespoons	=	1 cup or 8 ounces
2 cups	=	1 pint
2 pints	=	1 liquid quart
4 quarts	=	1 liquid gallon

❑

Canned Goods Weights & Measures

8 ounces	=	1 cup
10 1/2–12 ounces	=	1 1/4 cups
14–16 ounces	=	1 1/2 cups
16–17 ounces	=	2 cups
1 lb. 4 ounces	=	2 1/2 cups
1 lb. 13 ounces	=	3 1/2 cups

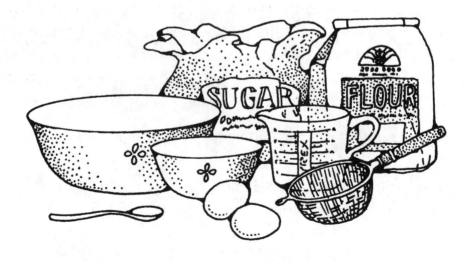

Keeping Food Safe to Eat Is Up to You

We live in a time when many people are suspicious, almost afraid, of their food. Some fears about the safety of our food supply are reasonable, and some are not. It's important to realize that most of the dangers associated with food are due to the way we handle it in our own kitchens. In the United States, about 9,000 people die from food poisoning every year.[4] Millions and millions of others have an uncomfortable few days with what they think is "stomach flu." Most of these illnesses could have been prevented through careful handling of food by the cook.

Food-borne illnesses are usually caused by bacteria. Some are caused by viruses or poisonous chemicals. We'll refer to bacteria and viruses together as *germs.*

Germs are found everywhere, in soil, air, animals' bodies (including ours), on fruits and vegetables, in milk . . . but before you swear you'll never eat or breathe again, realize that most aren't harmful to us (some are even helpful, like the bacteria that make yogurt). Others are only a problem if there are a lot of them around, or if they've had the chance to manufacture toxins that will hurt us even when the germs are dead. To survive, germs need:[5]

- food and water
- *time* to reproduce or make toxins
- the right *temperature*
- a way to get around (they can't wiggle into our custard by themselves, but they *can* hitchhike on our fingers)

So when we talk about preventing food poisoning, most of what we're dealing with involves giving the germs as little time as possible at the temperatures they like, so they can't do their dirty work. We also want to introduce as few bacteria as we can into our stew, or salad, in the first place. Food becomes unsafe to eat through six main boo-boos:

- poor personal hygiene on the part of people working with food
- preparing food that may already have been spoiled or contaminated by poisons

- storing food without proper care
- handling food carelessly
- using unclean equipment or working in a dirty kitchen
- allowing insects or rodents to infest food supplies

Food safety is *very* serious business. What follows might seem like an impossibly long list of guidelines for keeping food safe to eat. But every point in the list is crucial, so it's worth reviewing over and over until all of these practices are second nature to you.

Start With Personal Hygiene

- Always wash hands before you begin to handle food.
- Wash hands again after you:
  - use the toilet
  - change a child's diaper or assist a child in the bathroom
  - touch your face, hair, or any infected part of your body
  - blow your nose, sneeze, or cough
  - touch dirty rags, clothing, or work surfaces
  - clear away dirty dishes and utensils
  - touch raw food, especially meat, fish or poultry
  - handle money or smoke a cigarette
- Keep your fingernails clean and short.
- Avoid wearing rings (except a simple band), bracelets, and anything that would dangle into the food.
- Keep hair clean and long hair tied back.
- Wear clean clothing.
- Don't work with food when you're sick.
- Don't smoke in the kitchen.

THE

STOP DISEASE

METHOD OF
HAND WASHING

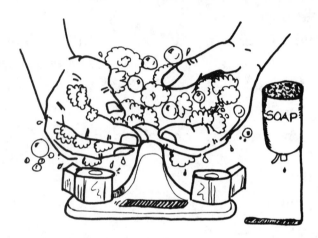

The following handwashing method should be used:

- Use liquid soap from a dispenser and running water
- Rub your hands vigorously as you wash them
- Wash all surfaces including:

    - backs of hands

    - wrists

    - between fingers

    - under fingernails

- Rinse your hands well with running water
- Dry your hands with a paper towel
- Turn off the water using a paper towel instead of bare hands
- Discard towel in covered trash can controlled by a foot pedal

Source: *Childhood Emergencies—What to Do, A Quick Reference Guide,* by Marin Child Care Council (formerly Project Care for Children), Bull Publishing Company.

Be Picky About the Foods You Serve

- ❑ Buy only from reputable stores or dealers.
- ❑ Don't buy or accept for delivery foods that look spoiled or infested with insects.
- ❑ Use only pasteurized milk.
- ❑ Don't serve home-canned foods to children you take care of.
- ❑ Don't serve raw eggs in any form (like eggnog) and don't allow children to taste items like raw cookie dough containing eggs.
- ❑ Don't serve spoiled or moldy foods, food from a bulging or leaky can, or anything else that looks or smells suspicious. If you have doubts, toss it, and don't take a little taste to test it! Some very dangerous foods taste OK.
- ❑ Pay attention to "use by" or "sell by" dates on food packages.

Store Foods Carefully

- ❑ Store foods at the right temperatures:

    Refrigerator: 32–40° F

    Freezer: 0° F or below

    Pantry: 65° or below is best

- ❑ Don't waste any time in getting perishable foods into the refrigerator or freezer after shopping or receiving a delivery.
- ❑ Stored foods should be dated, labeled if necessary, and kept off the floor.
- ❑ Place newer foods behind older ones in the storage area . . . "first in, first out."
- ❑ Don't store opened food in cans in the refrigerator. Transfer the food to glass or plastic containers.
- ❑ Cover all stored foods.
- ❑ Store cooked foods *above* raw foods in the refrigerator.
- ❑ Store foods separately from chemicals, cleaners, etc.

❏ Leave space for air circulation in the refrigerator. Don't line the shelves with foil. Keep it clean and check every day for food that should be tossed out. Check the thermometers in the refrigerator and freezer.

❏ Store packages of thawing meat or poultry in bowls or shallow pans so their juices can't drip on foods below.

❏ Leftovers should be kept in the refrigerator for no more than 72 hours.

Handle Food with Respect

❏ Keep perishable foods at safe temperatures. If they're to be eaten cold, keep them at 40°F or below. If they're supposed to be hot, they must be 140°F or above. If you aren't going to serve hot foods soon, refrigerate them in shallow pans. The center of the food must reach 45° or less within 4 hours. Don't leave perishable foods out on the counter while you're working on a recipe with many steps.

❏ Avoid touching foods with your hands. Use scoops, tongs, other utensils, and disposable gloves whenever possible.

❏ Wash fruits and vegetables thoroughly before using them.

❏ Thaw frozen foods in the refrigerator or in the microwave. Bacteria can be happily setting up colonies on the outside of the food even when the center is frozen.

❏ Cook fish, poultry, eggs, and meat thoroughly. Poultry should be cooked to an internal temperature of 180°F, meat to 160°F. Because of widespread salmonella contamination in eggs, we're not supposed to eat soft-cooked eggs any more.

❏ Taste those delicacies you're concocting with two spoons, the professional way. Spoon One goes into the food and then transfers it to Spoon Two (the spoons can't touch). Spoon Two goes into your mouth.

❏ Hold plates by the rims, drinking glasses by the bottoms, cups and silverware by the handles.

- ❏ Never serve food that's left on anyone's plate to another person.
- ❏ Don't mix leftover food and fresh-cooked food unless it's in good condition and the mixture will be used up immediately.
- ❏ Wipe the tops of cans before you open them.
- ❏ Don't serve or store foods in antique or imported pottery (especially from Mexico, China, Hong Kong, or India) unless it has been verified to be lead-free. Lead from the glazes can leak into food and has caused many cases of lead poisoning in the United States.[16]

Run a Clean Operation

- ❏ Don't allow animals or cat litter boxes in the kitchen.
- ❏ Regularly clean your equipment, kitchen, and eating area (see *The Squeaky-Clean Scrubbing Schedule*, page 150).
- ❏ Don't let anyone sit on counters or work surfaces.
- ❏ Keep rugs out of food preparation areas.
- ❏ Wash the can opener in between uses. It's one of the most overlooked sources of germs in the kitchen![7]
- ❏ Air-dry rather than towel-dry dishes and utensils.
- ❏ Clean any cutting board or utensil that has touched raw meat, poultry, or eggs before any other cooked or raw food comes in contact with it. Plastic cutting boards are the best because they don't provide housing areas for bacteria.
- ❏ Don't use cracked tableware or containers; bacteria can find food and a nice place to live in the cracks.
- ❏ Use freshly laundered towels and rags.
- ❏ Sanitize sponges occasionally with a bleach solution or run them through the dishwasher.

Don't Put Out the Welcome Mat for Insects and Rodents

❑ Keep your kitchen immaculate.

❑ Store opened packages of food within tightly sealed containers.

❑ Remove garbage promptly and keep the outdoor garbage area clean.

❑ Don't store food under the sink.

❑ Keep doors and windows tightly screened. When screens get holes, fix them.

❑ Caulk openings and cracks around sinks, drain pipes, and water pipes. Repair cracks in walls.

❑ Inspect containers and cardboard boxes that you bring into your building. Cockroaches, especially, like to hitchhike in them.

❑ If you notice some pests around, take care of the problem before it gets bigger. Should you find that you'll have to use an insecticide, follow the directions carefully.

CAUTION!!

These foods can be dangerous

Raw or undercooked meat, poultry, and fish

Raw milk

Raw or undercooked eggs

Cooked vegetables or grains left at room temperature for long periods of time

Raw shellfish

Homemade ice cream (with eggs)

Cooked foods containing eggs, such as custards and cream pies

Improperly canned low-acid foods, such as green beans, corn, spinach, mushrooms, olives, beets, asparagus, pork, beef, and seafood

---

The Squeaky-Clean Kitchen Scrubbing Schedule

We know that cleanup isn't usually the most attractive aspect of any job. A well-used kitchen can rapidly turn into a public health hazard, though, without conscientious cleaning. Then it's *really* no fun. The grime in a kitchen will never get out of hand if you set up a cleaning schedule and follow it. So here it is, preventive medicine for your kitchen:

Constantly

❑ Wipe up spills and splashes from:

- work surfaces
- floors
- walls
- range
- microwave
- refrigerator

❑ Wash equipment after each use:

- can opener
- mixer
- blender
- food processor

Daily

❑ Make sure all dishes, utensils, etc. are washed.

❑ Wipe down work tables and counters.

❑ Wipe down range, microwave, refrigerator, dishwasher.

❑ Sweep and damp mop kitchen floor.

❑ Take out the trash.

❑ Check refrigerator and freezer temperatures.

Weekly

❑ Scrub kitchen floor.

❑ Remove burners from range and clean underneath them.

❑ Clean the inside of the refrigerator. Throw out old food. A mixture of baking soda and water may be used to wipe the shelves and walls.

❑ Clean out the food trap in the dishwasher.

❑ Clean the filter from the smoke hood.

Saving Time in the Kitchen

If you're taking care of children by yourself, you know it's important to be supervising *them,* not a gourmet dish that's bubbling out of control on the stove. And even if you are in the position of primarily cooking for children, it's still nice to save time here are there so you can do other important things . . . like cleaning and equipment maintenance, bookwork, developing new recipes, and staff training. Here are some time-saving tips, learned the hard way during years of collective experience:

❏ Plan menus ahead of time, check for ingredients on hand, make a detailed shopping list, and shop only once a week.

❏ Remember that the children probably won't appreciate three elaborate menu items in a meal. *Keep it simple.* Skip the fancy sauces.

❏ It's OK to serve some cold foods, or even a full meal of them.

❏ Plan for leftovers that can show up later in another form. (Example: turkey loaf, served later on as a cold sandwich filling or as cubes on a snack tray).

❏ Do as much in one pot or pan as possible. Avoid recipes that lead to a tower of dirty dishes in the sink. See if you can revise your old favorites to save steps.

❏ Make larger portions than you need and freeze some for later. Casseroles, soups, sauces, and quick breads lend themselves readily to this.

❏ Do as much of the food preparation as possible when the children aren't around or are napping, unless you want to have them pitch in. You may find it works to set up an activity for them in the kitchen while you're doing certain phases of the food preparation.

❏ Use time-saving appliances like food processors, when they really will save time. Consider setup and cleanup time.

Safety for Adults in the Kitchen

Burns, cuts, and falls can put a damper on your fun in the kitchen. Don't let them happen to you! Follow these guidelines. . . .

- ❏ Allow yourself enough time for the job. Most accidents happen when you're in a hurry or aren't paying attention to what you're doing.
- ❏ Wipe up grease or wet spots and pick up loose items from the floor immediately.
- ❏ Don't run or allow running in the kitchen.
- ❏ Use a ladder if you're reaching for items stored on high shelves.
- ❏ If you can, store heavier items on lower shelves.
- ❏ Keep your knives sharp; you are more likely to be cut by a dull knife since you need to use more pressure.
- ❏ Store knives separately, not loose in a drawer with other utensils.
- ❏ Don't soak knives in a dishbasin; you could cut yourself reaching into the water.
- ❏ Make sure that your hands (and feet) are dry before plugging in or unplugging electrical appliances.
- ❏ Don't reach into a toaster with a metal utensil unless the toaster is unplugged.
- ❏ To unplug an appliance safely, turn it off, then hold the plug close to the electrical outlet and pull gently.
- ❏ Keep equipment in good repair. Be on the lookout for frayed cords and straining motors.
- ❏ Keep items that burn easily (pot holders, towels, curtains, billowy sleeves, and the like) away from burners and other sources of heat.
- ❏ Keep the oven and broiler cleaned regularly; grease buildup could lead to a fire.
- ❏ When cooking with a covered pan, take the lid off facing away from you to avoid being scalded.

Making a Kitchen Safe for Young Children

- ❏ Keep all poisonous products in locked cupboards.
- ❏ Keep all poisonous products in their original containers; don't transfer them into soda bottles or coffee cans.
- ❏ Use safety latches on cabinets.
- ❏ Keep potentially dangerous items like knives, matches, boxes with serrated edges, toothpicks, and plastic bags in one place, out of reach.
- ❏ Make sure that your drawers have safety catches so they don't crash to the floor when they're pulled out too far.
- ❏ When you're using the stovetop, keep pot handles turned toward the center of the stove.
- ❏ Watch out for appliance cords dangling over the counter. If you leave toasters, coffeemakers, etc., on the counter, unplug them when not in use, place them against the wall, and tuck the cords behind them.
- ❏ If you can, get a garbage disposal that only operates with a lid in place.
- ❏ Don't store alcoholic beverages, vitamins, and medicines in the refrigerator or any place accessible to a young child.
- ❏ Many children are burned by hot water from the tap. Supervise them closely at the sink.
- ❏ Teach children the proper way to use a knife (some don't realize which side of the blade is the cutting edge) and supervise always.
- ❏ Keep a first aid kit handy.
- ❏ Set aside child-safe kitchen equipment in a lower cabinet so the children can "play cooking" while you're working in the kitchen.

Using Your Microwave Safely

Since there is a wide array of models on the market, and because, with the speed of technology, new and different versions will be out each year, we recommend that you read the instructions that come with the microwave oven you are using and keep them handy for reference and service information.

Microwave ovens, when used and maintained properly, are considered to be extremely safe. There are some basic safety rules, however, that everyone who uses a microwave oven should know.

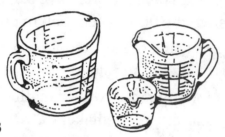

Important Safety Rules

❑ Follow the manufacturer's instructions for use.

❑ Keep the oven clean, especially around the door seal.

❑ Never tamper with any part of the oven.

❑ If you suspect any damage to the oven, be sure to call a qualified service person to check it out.

❑ Heat-proof glassware and glass-ceramic (Corning Ware type) cookware seem to be the best choices for use in the microwave, with round containers resulting in more even heating than square or rectangular ones. Here's how to test glass for microwave-cooking safety: Fill a glass measuring cup with one cup of water and put it in the microwave oven alongside of the container you are testing. (The cup of water is included because the oven should never be operated without food or liquid in it to absorb the energy.) Run the microwave oven on HIGH for one minute.

> *If the container stayed cool, it's okay to cook in it.*
> *If it was only lukewarm; it's okay to reheat in it;*
> *Don't use it in the microwave if it got warm.*[9]

- ❏ Always choose containers that are colorless and plain; color and decoration can interfere with the transmission of microwaves.[8]

- ❏ Other types of containers such as plastic yogurt or margarine tubs, *and even plastic containers that are marked "microwave-safe,"* may have chemical components that can "migrate" into the food at high temperatures.

- ❏ For the same reason, if you cover food with plastic wrap while cooking or heating, do not let the covering come in contact with the heating food. Also, be sure to use only the kind of plastic wrap which is recommended for use in the microwave, since other types can melt into the food.

- ❏ Avoid heat-susceptor packaging. At this time its safety has not been thoroughly established.[10,11]

- ❏ Recycled paper products should not be used in the microwave. They may contain small metal fragments which can set the paper on fire during cooking.

Preventing Microwave Burns

- ❏ Beware of microwave burns. The container or some portions of the food may be cool enough to touch while other portions may be hot enough to cause external or internal (mouth and esophagus) burns. Fats and sugars can get especially hot in the microwave and must be handled with extreme caution.

- ❏ Puncture foods that have unbroken skins, such as potatoes, tomatoes, sausage, etc., to allow steam to escape and prevent bursting. Do not cook eggs in the shell for the same reason.

- ❏ To prevent being burned by escaping steam, puncture plastic wrap if you are using it to cover the cooking food.

- ❏ Stay with the oven if you're popping popcorn. Heat buildup can cause a fire.

- ❏ Do not heat baby bottles in the microwave. Uneven heating may result in hot spots in the bottle which are not easily apparent, and can be quite dangerous.[12]

❏ Heating baby food in jars can cause the food to erupt out of the jar and can also result in uneven heating. If you heat baby food in the microwave, place it in a shallow container, stir it well after heating to equalize the heat, and *always test it first* to be sure the food is not too hot for the baby.

Preventing Food Poisoning

❏ Check to be sure food is thoroughly and evenly heated/cooked. Cold spots can harbor harmful bacteria which can cause food poisoning.

❏ Discard foods forgotten in the microwave if they were there for over two hours after thawing. Ordinary cooking won't destroy harmful bacteria that may have formed.

❏ Always cook meat, poultry and fish thoroughly. Use a microwave temperature probe or check with a meat thermometer to be sure meat is cooked to a safe temperature—at least 175°F. for pork, 180°F. for poultry. Check temperature in several places. After cooking it should be left to stand for 10–15 minutes under a foil tent to let temperatures equalize. Stuffing should be cooked separately to minimize chance of bacterial growth.

❏ Here are the agencies to contact if you need more information about microwave cooking safety:

- For questions about microwave ovens or packaging call the nearest U.S. Food & Drug Administration office listed in your phone book.

- For questions about cooking poultry and meat call the USDA food safety hot line at 1-800-535-4555 or (202) 447-3333 in the Washington D.C. area, or write to The Meat and Poultry Hotline, USDA-FSIS, Room 1165-S, Washington D.C. 20250.

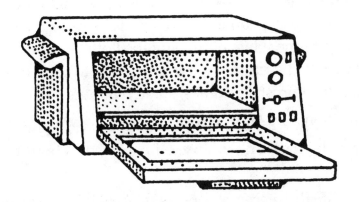

Miscellaneous Microwave Facts, Tips and Techniques

- ❑ Food cut into uniform size and shape will cook more evenly.

- ❑ Unevenly shaped food should be placed with the thickest part toward the outside of the baking dish.

- ❑ Since the amount of liquid in a food affects the cooking time, foods with more moisture will get hotter than foods that are drier (for example, when heating a sandwich the filling may get hotter than the bread). Remember to test different parts.

- ❑ When cooking a number of items, such as potatoes, place them in an evenly-spaced circle. This will allow air circulation and more even cooking.

- ❑ Stir, rearrange and rotate foods to achieve even cooking. This is especially important when making sauces.

- ❑ Many foods cooked in a microwave oven continue to cook for 5–20 minutes after the oven is off. Some recipes for microwave cooking include this time in the directions. This is an important part of the cooking process, especially for dense foods such as roasts.

- ❑ Do not sprinkle meat or vegetables with salt until after they're cooked. Salt will draw liquid out of the food and interfere with the cooking process.

❑ One great advantage of a microwave oven is that it's able to defrost food quickly. Use the defrost or low power so that the food will not begin to cook on the outside before thawing on the inside. Alternate equal times of standing time and microwaving time while defrosting to allow the heat to become evenly distributed without starting to cook the food. For example, defrost 5 minutes, stand 5 minutes, and so on.

❑ Some additional tips for defrosting:

- Covering the dish with waxed paper helps to diffuse the microwaves.

- Separate the pieces as soon as they thaw enough and rearrange them more evenly.

- As soon as possible, stir, chop up or rotate food.

- If some pieces thaw first, remove them while the others continue to thaw.

❑ To decrystallize honey or jam, remove the metal lid from the glass jar and microwave on HIGH for 1–2 minutes or until crystals have melted.

❑ Packages of tortillas can be softened and warmed by wrapping the number you need in paper towels and microwaving on high for 6–7 seconds per piece.

❑ For easier cutting of the tough outer skin of a hard winter squash, microwave it uncovered on HIGH for 1–2 minutes and then let stand for 1–2 more minutes before cutting.

❑ To reheat casserole-type leftovers, place covered, microwave-safe container in oven on HIGH for 2 minutes per cup of refrigerated food. Stop and stir after one minute.

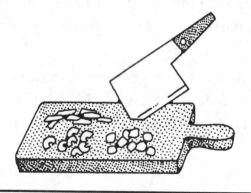

Children's Use of Microwave Ovens

It is a fact of modern life that children are frequent users of microwave ovens. (A 1988 study by Campbell Microwave Institute found 70% of children ages six to twelve using microwave ovens at home.)[13]

This clearly presents the potential for serious accidents. A study by Shriners Burns Institute in Cincinnati has documented an increased number of children scalded or burned by microwaved foods.[14] Here are some things to consider when assessing the ability of a child to use a microwave oven safely.

❏ Does the child have the ability to understand cause and effect, for example, "If I do this, then that will happen."?

❏ Can the child competently read, understand and follow directions?

❏ Is the child tall enough to easily remove food from the oven with both hands? Many of the serious burns reported have resulted from hot food spilling on the child who attempts to remove it from the oven.

❏ Is the child capable of understanding and upholding all of the safety rules listed on pages 154–156, *Using Your Microwave Safely*?

There is no age at which using any stove or oven is completely risk-free. However, the risk to children, simply due to their smaller size and limited experience, is likely to be greater than to adults. We strongly urge adults who decide to permit children to use microwave ovens (or any stove or oven), to do so with extreme caution, thorough explanation of safety rules and considerable practice in the presence of an adult. Here are a few additional safety tips if children will be using the microwave oven:

❏ Be sure that the oven is on a sturdy surface and can't be tipped.

❏ Have a table or counter nearby so that the cookware can be set down nearby immediately upon removing it from the oven.

❏ Be sure that the child always uses oven mitts to minimize the risk of burns. Portions of the dish may be hot or hot food may spill over the edge.

CHAPTER SEVEN

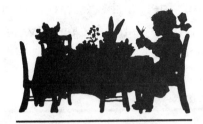

Environmental Concerns

Hints for an Earth-Friendly Kitchen

Each of us makes many choices every day that have an impact on the environment and affect the kind of world we're building for our children. With just a little thought and effort we can develop and maintain habits that contribute to a healthier planet. Try posting a reminder list in the kitchen of 3 or 4 earth-friendly improvements you are pretty sure you can make. When those become second nature, post a new list. What you do *does* make a difference.

To save water

- ❏ Wash dishes in a dishpan instead of under running water.
- ❏ Rinse the dishes with the faucet on halfway and only on while in use. (50% of wasted water in homes is due to letting the tap run unnecessarily.)[1]
- ❏ If you use a dishwasher, only run it when it is full.
- ❏ When peeling fruits or vegetables which will need to be washed, set them aside in a colander until they're all peeled, then wash them all at once.
- ❏ Fix leaky faucets right away. Even tiny leaks waste lots of water. Meanwhile, catch the drips in a container for watering plants.

- Use a low-flow aerator (available at most hardware stores) on your faucet.
- If you have a water meter, check it to find hidden leaks. (If there is a leak, it will register use even when all the water in the house is turned off.)

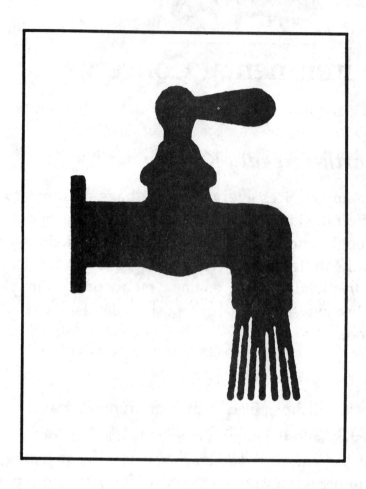

To save energy

- Use cold water instead of hot whenever possible.
- Keep a container of cold drinking water in the refrigerator to avoid having to let the faucet run until the water gets cold.
- Keep the refrigerator and freezer only as cold as you need to—refrigerator 32-40°; freezer 0°.
- Make sure the refrigerator door seal is tight.

❏ Periodically use a brush or vacuum to clean the condenser coils on the back of the refrigerator. (Unplug it while doing this.) Dirt and dust make it more difficult for the coils to stay cool.

❏ If you have a manual defrost freezer, defrost it regularly. Frost build-up causes the motor to run longer.

❏ Defrost frozen foods in the refrigerator—it will help keep the refrigerator cold, using less energy.

❏ Don't leave the refrigerator door open unnecessarily.

❏ For cooking small portions, pressure cookers, toaster ovens and microwave ovens are more energy efficient than conventional ovens. For large items such as turkeys, microwaving is the least efficient.[2]

❏ Only preheat the oven when it is really necessary, and then, for the shortest possible time. (Ten minutes is usually adequate.)

❏ Don't open the oven door while baking; you'll let a lot of heat escape. Use a timer and look through the oven window.

❏ Match the pot size to the burner, using the smallest of both for the job, and use lids on pots to speed up cooking.

❏ Use glass or ceramic baking dishes for baking—they retain heat well and you can lower the oven temperature 25°.

❏ Use compact fluorescent lighting instead of incandescent bulbs—they're 3 to 4 times more energy-efficient.[2]

❏ Insulate your hot water heater and accessible hot water pipes.

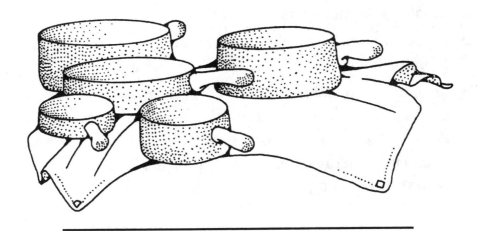

Planning a Kitchen for Energy Efficiency

If you are designing a new kitchen, or remodeling an existing one, you have a great opportunity to build energy efficiency right into your plans.

❑ Purchase energy-efficient appliances—check their federally mandated Energy Guide Labels to compare and rate them.

❑ Choose a refrigerator with a top freezer compartment rather than a side-by-side model, which uses up to 35% more energy.

❑ Choose a chest-type freezer over an upright if you have the space. They are 10-15% more energy-efficient. Also, an automatic defrost model consumes 40% more electricity than an equivalent size and style manual defrost model.

❑ Select a dishwasher with a built-in water heater. With an insulating water heating jacket for your hot water heater you will be able to keep your household water temperature lower (110-120°). The dishwasher will heat only the water needed to wash the dishes to the necessary 140°.

❑ Plan to install the dishwasher away from the refrigerator or freezer. If that's not possible, put insulation between them. Heat and moisture from the dishwasher makes the refrigerator or freezer use more energy.

❑ Purchase a gas range with electric ignition instead of a pilot light. You will be cutting gas consumption by about 40% a year.

❑ Choose a convection oven over a conventional one. You will be able to lower temperatures and shorten cooking times.

❑ Install a solar hot water system.

❑ Include a built-in recycling system that is designed to coordinate with local recycling requirements.

❑ Refer to David Goldbeck's book, *The Smart Kitchen: How to Design a Comfortable, Safe, Energy-Efficient and Environmentally Friendly Workspace.* Woodstock, NY: Ceres Press, 1989, and also to the other resources listed on page 232, to help you with your planning.

Think of Mother Earth When You're Shopping

Most of us have grown up during the "disposables" or "throw-away" generations. Now that we are faced with the dire consequences, we find ourselves struggling to change some very ingrained environmentally harmful habits. With less than 5% of the world's population, our nation generates 25% of its pollutants and more than 30% of its garbage.[6] Did you know that every day Americans throw out an average of 4 pounds of garbage *each*. That totals a *daily* garbage heap of 438,000 tons—enough to fill 63,000 garbage trucks![7] By becoming "green" consumers we can directly reduce the amount of waste.

Here's how to shop with ecology in mind:

- ❑ First and foremost—if you don't really need it, don't buy it!

- ❑ Choose reusable items over disposable items whenever possible.

- ❑ Be picky about packaging . . .
  - look for products that have minimal packaging
  - choose products packaged in recycled (look for the symbol) or recyclable materials, or in reusable containers
  - choose products packaged in materials that are most easily recyclable in your community
  - buy eggs in cardboard cartons rather than foam plastic
  - avoid purchasing anything in foam plastic
  - let the store manager know why you are making these choices
  - write or call the manufacturers and let them know why you've chosen to buy or not to buy their products (You can usually find their address and phone number on the container. Many companies list an 800 phone number for consumers.)

- ❑ Bring your own canvas or string bags with you when you shop.

- When you must use bags from the store, choose paper which can be recycled over plastic (most of which are neither biodegradable or recyclable). Reuse bags by bringing them the next time you shop.
- Read labels—try not to purchase products with harmful ingredients.
- Buy the large size or buy in bulk.
- When you do make purchases in recyclable containers, be sure to actually recycle them.
- Talk to your children about why you are making these choices; this will help them develop their own "ecology awareness."

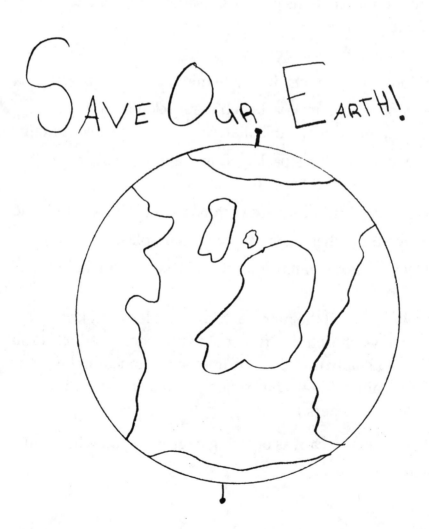

Making Everyone a Part of Your Recycling Plan

Whether its in the home or in the child care setting, establishing a recycling program works best if everyone is involved. Adults can take responsibility for gathering or purchasing necessary supplies and transporting wastes to the recycling center, older children can help with research, planning, set-up and maintenance of the program. Younger children can help by decorating boxes to use as storage containers and helping to decide where to keep them and by sorting recyclables.

Here are some ideas to help you establish a successful recycling program:

❏ Find out what local recycling programs are available in your community (see page 169 for state recycling phone numbers) and find out what items can be recycled.

❏ If you do not have a curbside pick-up program in your community, decide on a practical schedule for going to the recycling center.

❏ Decide on the most convenient place(s) to store the recyclables—kitchen, garage, back porch, closet, etc. If you don't have lots of space in a nearby, convenient spot (e.g., kitchen), use small containers there and, when full, empty them into larger bins in an outside storage area (e.g., basement). The more convenient your system, the quicker you will adapt to using it.

❏ Select containers, preferably with handles or on wheels, that won't be too heavy or bulky to carry when they fill up. Some possible choices: sturdy cardboard cartons, paper grocery bags, empty milk crates, plastic laundry baskets, rattan baskets, or recycling storage units specially designed for the purpose. (See *Appendix D—Resources* for places to order these.)

❏ As they accumulate, sort your recyclable items into the containers to be set out for curbside pick-up or delivered to the recycling center.

❏ If you have a yard, establish a compost for recycling food waste (other than meat products) and other organic materials.*

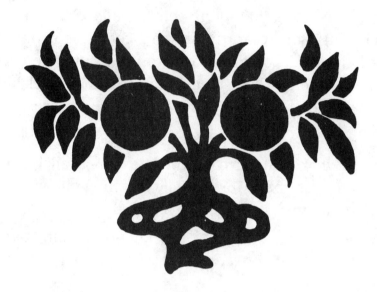

❏ Be creative about recycling items that can't be taken to the recycling center. Clothes and household goods that are in useable condition can be donated to non-profit organizations. Many items are usable for arts, crafts and science projects with children. A current fashion trend is jewelry, art pieces and clothing made of recycled material—a sign of the times!

❏ If there is no recycling program in your community, join with other concerned residents and get one started. *The Recycler's Handbook: Simple Things You Can Do,* by The Earthworks Group will tell you how to begin.

*To learn more about composting turn to page 176.

State Recycling Phone Numbers and Recycling Hotlines
Environmental Defense Fund
1-800-225-5333

Alabama: 205-271-7700
Alaska: 907-465-2666
Arizona: 602-255-3303
Arkansas: 501-562-7444
California: 916-323-3508
Colorado: 303-320-8333
Connecticut: 203-566-8895
Delaware: 302-736-5742
District of Columbia: 202-767-8512
Florida: 904-488-0300
Georgia: 404-656-3898
Idaho: 208-334-2789
Illinois: 217-782-6761
Indiana: 317-232-8883
Iowa: 515-281-3426
Kansas: 913-296-1500
Kentucky: 502-564-6716
Louisiana: 504-342-1216
Maine: 207-289-2111
Maryland: 301-974-3291
Massachusetts: 617-292-5962
Michigan: 517-373-0540
Minnesota: 612-296-8439
Minnesota: 612-536-0816
Mississippi: 601-961-5171

Missouri: 314-751-3176
Montana: 406-444-2821
Nebraska: 402-471-4210
Nevada: 702-885-4420
New Hampshire: 603-224-6996
New Jersey: 201-648-1978
New Mexico: 505-827-2780
New York: 518-457-7336
North Carolina: 919-733-7015
North Dakota: 701-224-2366
Ohio: 614-265-6353 or 614-644-2917
Oklahoma: 405-271-7519
Oregon: 503-229-5826
Pennsylvania: 717-787-7382
South Dakota: 605-773-3153
Tennessee: 615-741-3424
Texas: 512-458-7271
Utah: 801-538-6170
Vermont: 802-244-8702
Virginia: 804-786-8679
Washington, DC: 202-939-7116
West Virginia: 304-348-3370
Wisconsin: 608-267-7565
Wyoming: 307-777-7752

State Recycling Hotlines

Alabama: 1-800-392-1924
California: 1-800-RECYCAL
Colorado: 1-800-438-8800
Delaware: 1-800-CASHCAN
Maryland: 1-800-345-BIRP
Minnesota: 1-800-592-9528
New Jersey: 1-800-492-4242

Ohio: 1-800-282-6040
Rhode Island: 1-800-RICLEAN
Tennessee: 1-800-342-4038
Texas: 1-800-CLEANTX
Virginia: 1-800-KEEPITT
Washington: 1-800-RECYCLE

Source: *The Green Lifestyle Handbook,* Jeremy Rifkin, Editor, Henry Holt & Company, New York,1990.

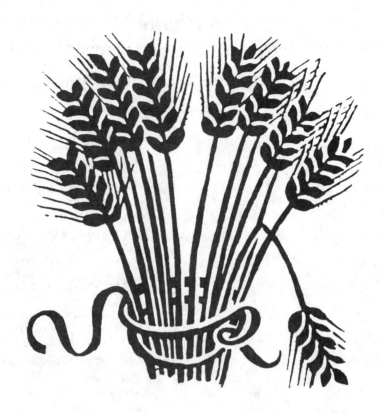

Homemade and Nontoxic Cleaning Products

What's a safe and economical way to keep your home and center squeaky-clean? You can make your own non-toxic cleaning products.

Many of the commercial household cleaning products that we have become accustomed to using are composed of harsh, toxic chemicals that add to environmental pollution and may also be harmful to our skin and lungs. (The average American home uses approximately 25 gallons of hazardous chemicals per year![8]) When you purchase cleaning products, read labels and avoid buying products that include harmful ingredients (required by law to have some type of warning label or hazard symbol).

Examples of some of the more common and familiar hazardous substances included in cleaning products are ammonia, which is harmful to the skin, eyes and lungs; *chlorine bleach* which can be highly irritating to eyes, nose, throat and lungs, and *can result in deadly fumes if accidently mixed with ammonia;* and cresol, an ingredient in many disinfectants, which can cause poisoning by ingestion and inhalation.[9]

More and more companies are responding to consumer demands for environmentally safe products. With a bit of kitchen chemistry you can make your own safe and effective alternative cleaners, too.

Here are some cleaning products for you to try. The ingredients can be found in your grocery or hardware store or pharmacy.

General All-Purpose Cleaners

❑ Mix equal parts of white vinegar and water for general cleaning.

❑ Mix 3 tablespoons washing soda with 4 cups warm water. Rinse with clean water.

❑ Mix vinegar and salt together for a good surface cleaner.

❑ Dissolve 4 tablespoons baking soda in 1 quart warm water or use baking soda on a damp sponge to clean and deodorize surfaces. Baking soda can also be made into a paste and used with an old toothbrush to clean tile grout.

Disinfectants

❑ Mix 1/2 cup borax with 1 gallon hot water. Use on a sponge or cloth to disinfect kitchen and/or bathroom surfaces.

❑ Hydrogen Peroxide will disinfect surfaces.

❑ Isopropyl alcohol wiped on surfaces and allowed to dry is another effective disinfectant.

Dishwashing Soaps

❑ Use any phosphate-free dishwashing liquid.

❑ Use pure bar soap rubbed on a cloth or sponge.

Scouring Powders

❑ Sprinkle baking soda, borax, table salt or washing soda on any surface where you would normally use a scouring powder. Scrub with a damp cloth or plastic mesh scrubber and rinse.

Oven Cleaners

❑ Sprinkle water and then lots of baking soda in the oven. Scrub with steel-wool pads and more water as needed.

❑ To maintain an already reasonably clean oven, mix 2 tablespoons non-phosphate dishwashing liquid soap with 1 tablespoon borax in a spray bottle and fill with warm water. Spray the solution in the oven and leave for 20 minutes or more before wiping clean. Spread newspapers on the floor to catch drips.

Silver Polish

❑ Apply a paste of baking soda mixed with water. Then rub, rinse and dry the silver.

❑ Line the bottom of the kitchen sink with a sheet of aluminum foil. Fill with hot water and add 1/4 cup of baking soda, rock salt or table salt. Put the silver into the water for 2–3 minutes, then wash in soapy water and dry.

❑ Use toothpaste on an old toothbrush to remove tarnish from crevices. Rinse with warm water and polish with a soft cloth or chamois.

Brass and Copper Polish

❑ Use lemon juice or a slice of lemon sprinkled with baking soda. Rub with a soft cloth, rinse and dry.

Glass Cleaner

❑ Mix equal parts white vinegar and water in a spray bottle. Spray on window or mirror and dry with crumpled newspaper.

Drain Cleaner

- ❑ Prevent clogging by keeping a drain strainer over the sink drain and never pour grease down the drain. Pour a pot of boiling water down the drain once or twice a week.

- ❑ For clogged drains, first try a plunger or a mechanical snake. If it's still clogged, pour 1/2 cup salt and 1/2 cup baking soda down the drain, followed by 6 cups of boiling water. Let it sit for several hours before flushing with more water.

- ❑ Another formula for clearing clogged drains is to pour 1/2 cup of white vinegar and a handful of baking soda down the drain and cover it tightly for 1 minute. Then rinse with hot water.

Air Freshener

- ❑ Simmer vinegar or herb mixtures or spices (e.g., cinnamon sticks, cloves, etc.) in water.

Furniture Polish

- ❑ Use plain mayonnaise, straight from the jar. Rub on the wood with a soft cloth.

- ❑ Mix 2 parts olive oil with 1 part lemon juice.

- ❑ Mix 3 parts olive oil with 1 part white vinegar.

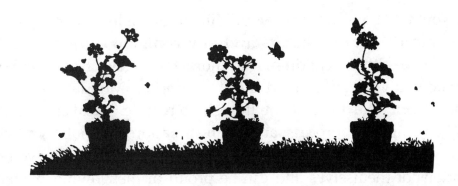

Source: Debra Lynn Dadd, *Nontoxic & Natural: How to Avoid Dangerous Everyday Products and Buy or Make Safe Ones* , Jeremy P. Tarcher, Inc., Los Angeles, 1984 and Debra Lynn Dadd, *The Nontoxic Home,* Jeremy P. Tarcher, Inc., Los Angeles, 1986.

Setting Goals and Making Changes, or "Every Little Bit Helps"

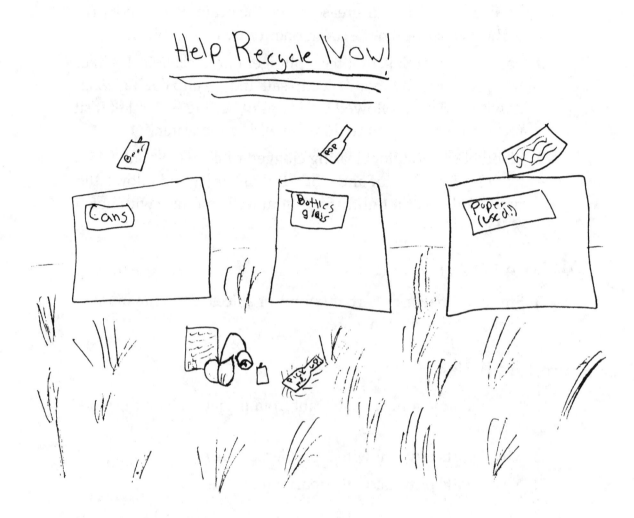

Well, if you're like we are, you would like to make lots of changes for the better—improve eating habits and environmental habits, add new activities to do with the children, read more, take a few classes, and on and on. Maybe you've even decided that "Starting on Monday I'll never use sugar again," or "Next month we'll begin to recycle." Realistically, change is usually a long slow, process, and taking an approach that acknowledges this fact is likely to result in more success. Also, adults who have realistic expectations of themselves and can be proud of their own achievements, even the small ones, will be able to have the same patient, supportive attitude toward the children they care for.

Some guidelines:

❏ Set only small achievable goals, and if you discover they weren't small enough, adjust them so that you will succeed. Remind yourself that any positive change is a plus. If you recycle a little, it's better than not at all. If you cut down a bit on fat and sugar, you're heading in the right direction.

❏ Incorporate health and environmental changes into your life through activities that you do anyway, such as: buying ecologically sound alternatives to products you usually use, or adding one new healthy recipe to your menu plan each week.

❏ When you are doing things that are good for your health and for the environment, talk about them matter-of-factly with the children. Each time we describe our actions to children we are helping to instill or strengthen awareness. They will be learning "why's" without a lecture.

❏ Acknowledge efforts that children make to be environmentally sensitive. Let them know that you notice and appreciate what they do. Perhaps the next generation will consider environmental abuses socially unacceptable.

❏ We adults know how hard it can be to change our old ways. Make the most of children's natural flexibility and adaptability. Let's help the next generation learn healthy, responsible habits from the beginning.

Build changes into your life gradually and patiently and before you know it new habits will become second nature.

Building a Compost Heap

Composting is a great way to help children learn the benefits of recycling organic garbage. The size of your compost will depend on how much space you have.

What to Do

- ❏ Choose an out-of-the-way spot in your yard, preferably a level, well-drained, sunny spot, but a shady one will work too. A 3' × 3' plot is a good size to retain heat and compost faster, but use whatever size space you have. **If you don't have a large enough dirt area, you can use a planter box.**

- ❏ A simple compost bin can be enclosed with chicken wire fencing formed into a cylinder or into a square by attaching it to four metal or wood posts.

- ❏ Line the bottom with moist peat moss, shredded paper, leaves or grass clippings. Sprinkle lightly with water as you add the layers.

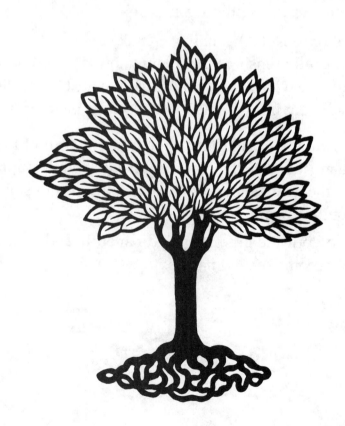

- Buy some earthworms at a local nursery or bait shop and put them into the compost mixture. Their continual tunneling helps to build rich and fertile soil and insure a successful compost.

- As you accumulate them, keep adding any food scraps (other than meat or dairy products) and other organic substances such as wood chips or garden clippings. High nitrogen substances such as blood meal, bone meal and manure can also be added to speed up the decaying process.

- Turn the mixture with a pitchfork or shovel every few days. Keep food scraps covered with grass clipping, dirt or leaves to avoid flies.

- Talk with the children about the changes taking place as you tend the compost together. Observe the worms at work. They're fun to watch and can help children learn respect for the value of all living things and the jobs they do.

- When the compost is broken down and ready to use, usually in two to eight weeks, dig in with the children and add your new "homemade" soil to the vegetable garden, around bushes and trees and to potted plants. If you sift it, you can use it as a planting mixture for sprouting garden seeds.

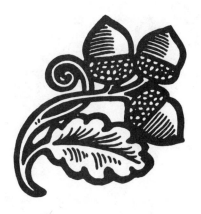

APPENDIX A

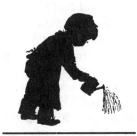

Nutrition Basics

The Basics of Good Nutrition

❏ *Nutrition* is the science concerned with food and how it is used by the body. It is also the combination of processes by which a person eats, digests, absorbs, utilizes, and excretes food substances.

❏ Nutrition is a young science—the first vitamin was discovered about 65 years ago, and we assume that more nutrients will be discovered in years to come. There are over 40 known nutrients, and no one food contains them all.

❏ *Nutrients* are the substances found in food that work together to provide energy, promote growth, and regulate body processes. The six major classes of nutrients are:

Carbohydrates	Vitamins
Proteins	Minerals
Fats	Water

Proteins, fats, and carbohydrates provide calories, which are small units of energy your body can use to do its work or stay warm.

The charts on pages 182–184 describe briefly the functions and good food sources of the major nutrients.

❏ Everyone has different nutritional needs, which depend upon age, sex, body size, heredity, activity levels, state of health, and even climate! Although more information is becoming available, we still don't know for certain what all of those needs are.

❏ Some nutrients are needed in large quantities and some in small. In the United States, nutrient requirements are sometimes expressed as *Recommended Dietary Allowances, or RDA.* The RDA are based upon the best available scientific research (they're updated every ten years or so), and they're supposed to cover the needs of almost all healthy people.

It's important for you to understand that the RDA aren't all that helpful for measuring the quality of an individual's diet. Suppose that someone ingested just 50% of his RDA for vitamin C one day. We couldn't necessarily assume that he is suffering from a vitamin C deficiency! Maybe his body only needs 25% of the RDA. But then again, he might need 95% of the RDA (unfortunately, human beings aren't born with owner's manuals, so we don't really know how much of each nutrient will make each person's body work best). What would be fair to say is that if this fellow habitually got about 50% of the RDA for vitamin C, he would have a greater **risk** of a deficiency than someone who took in 100% of the RDA.

For this reason it's a good idea to aim for food patterns that supply nutrients in quantities close to the Recommended Dietary Allowances. These allowances are quite helpful in planning "diets" for groups of people.[1] You can use them to check your menus for nutritional adequacy, but more on that later . . .

❑ While it is true that some people in the United States don't get enough of certain nutrients, it is far more common for us to get too *much* of others, namely fat, sugars, and sodium. Excessive intakes of these substances, along with a lack of fiber, are related to the "diseases of affluence" that kill millions and millions of Americans: heart disease, high blood pressure, diabetes, and cancer.

❑ Now, it might seem overwhelming to plan a diet that supplies all of the nutrients in the right amounts, but there are some tools that simplify the job. The *"Basic Four"* is one such tool (remember this from sixth-grade health class?); several servings from each of the following groups are recommended daily:

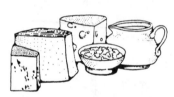

Milk and Dairy Foods

These foods supply calcium, protein, riboflavin, vitamin A, vitamin D, vitamin B_{12} and phosphorus.

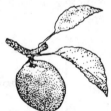

Fruits and Vegetables

Fruits and vegetables are sources of vitamin A, vitamin C, iron, vitamin B_6, folacin, and fiber.

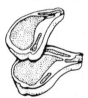

Meats and Meat Alternatives

Foods in this group are good sources of protein, iron, the B vitamins, and magnesium.

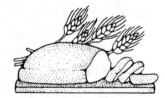

Breads and Cereals

You will find the B vitamins, minerals (especially iron), and fiber (if you use whole grains) in this group of foods.

Fats and *sweets* are sometimes called "extra foods," with no recommended number of servings—moderation is the key.

❏ Now, the Basic Four is certainly a useful guide, especially since most of us don't want to walk around with calculators to make sure that we're getting our RDA for every nutrient . . . but it is possible to meet the Basic Four guidelines and still be badly nourished. This is particularly likely to occur if the foods chosen are high in fat, salt, and/or sugar, are limited in their variety, or have been stored or prepared in ways that cause nutrients to be lost.

This issue has been clarified somewhat in the *Dietary Guidelines for Americans,* issued jointly by the US Department of Agriculture and the Department of Health and Human Services in 1990.[2] The Dietary Guidelines don't give us hard numbers, but they do steer us in the right direction, from a health promotion standpoint.

Dietary Guidelines for Americans

- Eat a variety of foods.
- Maintain healthy weight.
- Choose a diet low in fat, saturated fat, and πcholesterol.
- Choose a diet with plenty of vegetables, fruits, and grain products.
- Use sugars in moderation.
- Use salt and sodium in moderation.
- If you drink alcoholic beverages, do so in moderation.

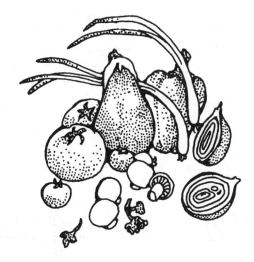

A User-Friendly Guide to Some Major Nutrients

Nutrients	Primary Functions	Rich Food Sources
Energy Nutrients (supply calories)		
Proteins	Supply amino acids to be used for growth and maintenance of the body	Meat, poultry, fish, eggs, milk, cheese, dried beans, tofu, peanut butter
*Carbohydrates**	Primary source of energy for the body's activities	*Complex carbohydrates:* breads, cereals, rice, pasta, tortillas, potatoes *Sugars:* sugar, honey, jelly, molasses, candy, milk, fruits
Fats	Provide energy, cushion vital organs, and supply essential fatty acids that maintain skin and membranes	Oils, butter, margarine, meat, lard, cream, olives, coconut, avocadoes, nuts

---

Fat Facts

Fats are made up of different combinations of fatty acids. These fatty acids may be saturated (solid at room temperature) or mono- or polyunsaturated (liquid at room temperature). Saturated fats are the ones that raise blood cholesterol. They are *usually* found in animal foods, like meat or milk (palm oil and coconut oil are two vegetable oils that are highly saturated, however).

Cholesterol is found only in foods of animal origin. It is possible for a food to have no cholesterol in it but still be very high in fat (and calories!). Corn oil, for example, is cholesterol-free but 100% fat.

---

*Fiber is also a carbohydrate, but it can't be digested by humans, so it provides bulk or "roughage" and no calories. Good sources are whole grains, fresh fruits and vegetables, dried fruits, dried beans.

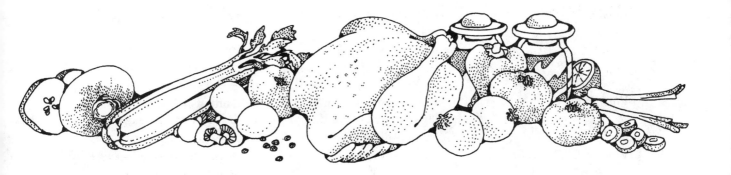

Nutrients	Primary Functions	Rich Food Sources
Water-Soluble Vitamins		
Thiamin (B₁)	Helps the body use carbohydrates for energy; important for health of nervous system	Pork, organ meats, yeast, eggs, green leafy vegetables, whole or enriched grains, dried beans
Riboflavin (B₂)	Helps the body get energy from carbohydrates, fats, and proteins; important for healthy mucous membranes	Milk, organ meats, yeast, cheese, eggs, green leafy vegetables, whole or enriched grains
Niacin	Helps the body release energy from foods; promotes healthy skin, digestive tract, and nervous system	Liver, yeast, whole or enriched grains, beef, pork, peanuts
Vitamin B₆	Helps the body use proteins and fats, keeps nervous system healthy	Yeast, whole grains, fish, poultry, meats, bananas, green leafy vegetables
Vitamin B₁₂	Helps the body make its genetic material, vital for health of nerve tissue	Meat, poultry, fish, eggs, milk products, a few specially fortified plant foods
Vitamin C	Helps form collagen, keep bones, teeth, and blood vessels healthy, antioxidant	Citrus fruits, tomatoes, peppers, potatoes, cantaloupe, strawberries, cabbage

Nutrients	Primary Functions	Rich Food Sources
Fat-Soluble Vitamins		
Vitamin A	Helps in growth and maintenance of skin and membranes, needed for healthy eyes and night vision	Liver, cream, egg yolk, butter, fortified dairy products, green, orange, and yellow vegetables and fruits
Vitamin D	Helps form and maintain bones and teeth, aids in calcium absorption	Fatty fish, liver, eggs, butter, fortified dairy foods
Vitamin E	Helps form red blood cells and other tissues, protects fatty acids and vitamin A	Vegetable oils, wheat germ, whole grains, liver, green leafy vegetables
Vitamin K	Needed for normal blood clotting	Cabbage, cauliflower, liver, vegetable oils, green leafy vegetables
Minerals		
Calcium	Builds and maintains bones and teeth, needed for blood clotting and muscle contraction	Milk products, fish eaten with bones, dried beans, broccoli, bok choy, collards, kale, blackstrap molasses
Iron	Forms components of blood that carry oxygen to cells	Liver, meat, dried beans, dried fruits, fortified cereal
Fluoride	Keeps bones and teeth strong	Fluoridated water, tea, sardines
Iodine	Part of thyroid hormones	Seafood, iodized salt, seaweed
Water (the most important nutrient)	An essential component of the body's structure, a solvent, transports nutrients and wastes, regulates body temperature	Beverages and most solid foods

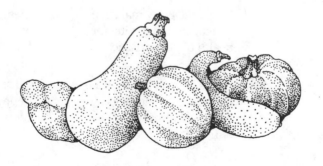

How Can You Tell Whether a Child is Getting Proper Nutrition?

A physician or registered dietitian is in the best position to judge whether a child is truly well-nourished, but in general, you can feel reasonably assured that a child is getting the nutrition she needs if she is growing well, is vigorous, and seems to have good resistance to illness (of course, most children will have occasional colds or bouts with flu). There are other indicators of good nutrition as well.[3] A child who is well-nourished will have:

- ❏ Erect posture and straight arms and legs (excepting infants)
- ❏ Good muscle tone
- ❏ Smooth skin, slightly moist, and with good color
- ❏ Good attention span, normal reflexes, psychologically stable
- ❏ Good appetite, normal elimination
- ❏ Normal heart rate and rhythm, normal blood pressure
- ❏ Normal sleeping habits
- ❏ Shiny hair, firmly rooted, and healthy scalp
- ❏ Smooth, moist lips
- ❏ Smooth, red tongue, not swollen
- ❏ Gums with a good pink color, no swelling or bleeding
- ❏ Teeth that are clean and free of cavities, well-shaped jaw
- ❏ Bright, clear eyes with healthy pink membranes
- ❏ Firm nails with pink nailbeds

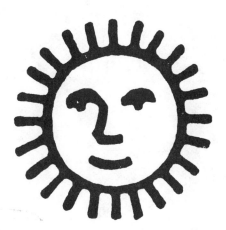

We do not recommend that you take it upon yourself to get into the medical diagnosis business, but you can alert families to signs that professional evaluation and treatment might be in order. Obviously, not all of these criteria are appropriate to use in the case of some children with physically handicapping conditions.

APPENDIX B

Special Topics

Allergies to Foods

Depending upon whom you believe, 0.3% to 38% of all children have food *allergies.*[1] In some cases, food allergies are only minor inconveniences. But they can also cause chronic health complaints, and in extreme cases, life-threatening reactions.

Food allergies are hard to diagnose, and even the most respected allergy specialists disagree about the best methods to use.[2] They also disagree on the range of health conditions that can be caused by allergies. Eczema, asthma, colic, migraine headaches, and hyperactivity have been linked to food allergies by some researchers, but not all.[3]

We do know that symptoms of food allergies usually appear in the first year of a child's life and often disappear within nine months or less.[4] And we also know that children are much more likely to have food allergies if their parents do (though not always to the same foods!).[3]

In a true food allergy, the body's immune system reacts to contact with the offending substance (*allergen*) by making *antibodies.* Through a series of mechanisms in the tissues of the body, symptoms are produced that may include:[1]

❏ hives   ❏ coughing

❏ vomiting   ❏ swelling of the throat

❏ eczema   ❏ nasal congestion

❏ diarrhea   ❏ wheezing

❏ sneezing   ❏ anaphylactic shock

A reaction can take from a few minutes to several days to occur.[3] The severity of the reaction can depend upon:

❏ how much of the allergen was eaten

❏ how often the food was eaten

❏ physical or emotional stress[2]

The foods most likely to cause allergies in children are: cow's milk, wheat, eggs, and corn. Soy products, oranges, chocolate, peanuts, legumes, rice, fish, beef, pork, and chicken are other potential allergens.[1]

Children can also have **sensitivities** or **intolerances** to foods. These are often confused with allergies. Examples are lactose intolerance, which is the inability to digest the sugars in milk, or sensitivities to food colorings and MSG.[2]

A child should have a professional evaluation when food allergies are suspected. It's a shame when a child is forced to avoid enjoyable foods that may not even be a problem for her. It's also a shame when a child suffers unnecessarily from allergy-related symptoms.

Be aware that allergies are not to be taken lightly, and can result in some troublesome situations:[5]

❑ Children can develop aversions to eating when they've been scared by severe allergic reactions or when restrictions make mealtimes unpleasant.

❑ Highly restrictive diets can be boring; they can also lead to serious nutrient deficiencies if they aren't well-planned.

❑ Children may use eating "forbidden" foods, or not eating at all, to manipulate their parents or caregivers.

Guidelines for Managing Food Allergies in Child Care

❑ Establish a written policy on parent/caregiver responsiblities in allergic conditions.

❑ Have a physician's statement on file which describes the allergy and recommended substitutions.

❑ Make sure a list of children with allergies and their "forbidden" foods is readily available for any adult who might be involved in preparing food or serving it to children.

❑ If a child is subject to life-threatening reactions from foods, obtain authorization to administer the appropriate medications and the necessary training to do so safely.

> **Anaphylactic shock can be fatal! Its warning signs are[2]**
>
> - itching and flushing of the skin
> - severe nausea or diarrhea
> - swelling of the respiratory passages

❑ Children with multiple food allergies, or allergies to foods that are primary sources of nutrients (as milk is in the United States), should be monitored by a physician or dietitian. Parents and caregivers may wish to receive counseling together regarding appropriate food choices.

❑ Be matter-of-fact about a child's food restrictions. Let the child take increasing responsibility for his food selections, as his awareness of what must be avoided grows. Tell other children in the group why the restrictions are necessary; hopefully they'll be supportive of their peer.

❑ Remember that children generally hate being singled out. Become adept at planning menus that everyone can eat, and when you find that you must make substitutions for a child, be sure that what she gets is as nice as what everyone else is getting. Don't make it too spectacular, though, or you'll have everyone else clamoring for that special treatment! (We recall one preschool classroom that was disrupted every lunch hour for weeks when a child's mother brought him fast-food chicken nuggets as his "allergy-free" lunch. Needless to say, none of the other children were interested in the standard menu).

❑ Become thoroughly familiar with foods that potentially contain the allergens you're avoiding. Read labels like crazy. Beware of "hidden" allergens in foods.

❑ Make every effort to replace the nutrients that will be missing when a child must avoid major foods and food groups. For example, apple juice is not a substitute for milk. Sure, they're both beverages, but apple juice has virtually none of milk's protein, calcium, riboflavin, vitamin A, or vitamin D.

Check the *Appendix D—Resources* for allergy cookbooks and suppliers of specialty foods.

Milk Allergies

Foods or ingredients to avoid

milk	casein
cheese	caseinate
cottage cheese	whey
yogurt	lactalbumin
butter	sodium caseinate
margarine with milk solids	lactose
milk chocolate	cream
creamed foods	calcium caseinate
custards and puddings	nonfat milk solids

Substitutes

soy milk	nut milks
soy formulas	juices, in baked goods
tofu	broth, in sauces or soups

Alternative food sources of important nutrients

Protein: meats, poultry, fish, eggs, dried beans, peanut butter

Calcium: spinach, collards, kale, turnip greens, broccoli, bok choy, soybeans, tofu (made with calcium sulfate), mustard greens, canned salmon with bones (they're soft!), corn tortillas, blackstrap molasses

Riboflavin: mushrooms, beet greens, spinach, broccoli, romaine lettuce, bok choy, asparagus, dried peaches, bean sprouts, fortified cereals

Egg Allergies

Foods or ingredients to avoid

eggs
some egg substitutes
mayonnaise
some salad dressings
egg noodles
most fresh pasta
custards, tapioca pudding

meringues
many baked goods
many breaded/batter-fried
   items
albumin
egg whites
egg yolks

Substitutes in recipes

Ener-G Egg Replacer®
extra 1/2 teaspoon baking
   powder for each egg missing
most dried pasta

arrowroot powder as a binder
tofu for pudding-like texture—
   can be "scrambled" too

Alternative food sources of important nutrients

Protein: meats, poultry, fish, dairy products, dried beans, nut butters
Vitamin A: fortified milk and margarine, yellow/orange and green leafy fruits and vegetables

Citrus Allergies

Alternative sources of vitamin C

cantaloupe, papaya, strawberries, green peppers, broccoli, cabbage, chiles, tomatoes, potatoes

Wheat Allergies

Foods or ingredients to avoid

wheat
wheat germ
wheat bran
modified food starch
graham flour
farina
semolina
gluten
vegetable starch
vegetable gum
enriched flour

Postum, malted milk
most baked goods
most crackers
macaroni, spaghetti
noodles
gravies, cream sauces
fried food coating
most baking mixes
soy sauce
some hot dogs, sausages
some salad dressings

Substitutes in recipes

cornstarch, tapioca,
   rice flour as thickeners
wheat-free breads, crackers
rice cakes
corn tortillas
oatmeal
polenta
cream of rice

wheat-free pasta
popcorn
rice flour
barley flour
potato flour
oat bran
rice bran
wheat-free cereal crumbs

Alternative food sources of important nutrients

Complex carbohydrates, B-vitamins, fiber: other whole grains . . . corn, barley, millet, rice, oats; potatoes, dried beans

Soy Allergies

Foods or ingredients to avoid

soybeans
soy flour
soybean oil
soy protein isolate
texturized vegetable
   protein (TVP)
vegetable starch
vegetable gum
tofu

soy sauce
teriyaki sauce
Worcestershire sauce
soy milk
soy infant formulas
some margarines
soy nuts
tempeh
miso

Corn Allergies

Foods or ingredients to avoid

cornmeal
corn starch
masa harina
corn oil
corn syrup
corn sweetener
vegetable starch
vegetable gum

some baked goods
some baking powder
corn tortillas
corn chips
some cold cereals
pancake syrups
many candies

Substitutes in recipes

other flours
potato starch, rice flour
   arrowroot, tapioca as
   thickeners
beet or cane sugar

pure maple syrup
baking soda and cream of
   tartar for leavening
honey
wheat flour tortillas

Anemia and Iron Deficiency

Normally oxygen is carried to the body's tissues as part of a molecule called *hemoglobin* in the red blood cells. When there's not enough hemoglobin around, a condition called anemia is the result. Most anemia is caused by *iron deficiency.* Iron deficiency anemia is the most common nutritional problem in the United States, affecting primarily children 12 to 36 months old, teenage boys, and women of childbearing age.[6] Iron deficiency anemia is found among children of all income levels, although it is more common in children from poorer families.[7,8]

Iron deficiency, even before outright anemia shows up, can have serious effects on the body's functioning. Infants with iron deficiency appear fearful, tense, unresponsive to examiners, and generally "unhappy."[8] Older children with mild iron deficiency have exhibited:

❏ a shortened attention span

❏ irritability

❏ fatigue

❏ inability to concentrate on tasks

❏ poor performance on vocabulary, reading, math, problem-solving, and psychological tests

❏ lowered resistance to infection[7]

How heartbreaking that children may do poorly in school, or be labeled "lazy" or "unmanageable," when in fact they are suffering from a preventable nutritional problem!

Iron deficiency can have several causes: a diet that's lacking in good sources of iron; poor absorption of iron in the intestines; increased requirements for iron, particularly during periods of rapid growth; heavy or persistent losses of blood; and some infections.[9] When young children become iron-deficient, it's often because they didn't get enough iron during their first year of life,[6] or because they've been consuming too much milk and not enough iron-rich foods.[10]

What You Can Do to Prevent Iron Deficiency

- Give infants **iron-fortified formula** or **breastmilk** up to the age of one year. Breastfeeding mothers may want to discuss iron supplementation with their pediatricians.

- When feeding cereal to infants who are between 4 to 6 months and one year old, use **iron-fortified infant cereals.**

- Serve children **iron-rich foods** frequently, at snacks as well as at meals. Organ meats, shellfish, and muscle meats are the richest sources of highly absorbable iron; don't feed liver more than once a week, though, or vitamin A toxicity can result. Nuts, green vegetables, whole grains, enriched breads and fortified cereals, and dried fruits are also good sources of iron.[1]

- The iron in non-meat foods is absorbed better when meats or **vitamin C-rich foods** are served at the same meal. Dairy products, eggs, and tea hinder the absorption of non-meat iron.[1]

- Don't allow children to fill up on milk and ignore other foods. A pint of milk a day is plenty for children after their first year, until they're teenagers.

Choking on Food

Every five days, a child in the United States dies from choking on food. Young children lack the chewing skills to deal with foods that are hard or tough. Also, foods that are round or sticky can block their airways, which are smaller than those of adults.

Although children have been known to choke on apple pieces, peanut butter sandwiches, cookies, carrots, popcorn, beans, and bread, the four foods that have caused the most deaths are:

- ❑ hot dogs
- ❑ nuts
- ❑ hard candy
- ❑ grapes[11]

Every adult who takes care of children should be aware of the simple precautions that can drastically reduce the risk of choking.

Choking Prevention

- **Always** supervise children while they are eating.
- Insist that children eat calmly and while they're sitting down. Encourage them to chew their food well.
- Infants should be fed solid foods only while they're sitting up.
- Make sure that the foods you serve the children are appropriate for their chewing and swallowing abilities. Do not give the following foods (unless they're modified . . . see page 59) to children younger than 4 years of age:
  - hot dogs
  - nuts
  - grapes
  - hard candies
  - hard pieces of fruits or vegetables
  - popcorn
  - peanut butter
- Don't allow children to eat in the car or bus; if a child started choking it might be hard to get the vehicle to the side of the road safely.[12,13]

CHOKING

CHOKING (when conscious)

Infant (birth to 1 year)

1. Supporting infant's head and neck, straddle over forearm, with head lower than trunk, and administer 4 back blows, high, between the shoulder blades. *(Fig. 1)*

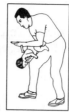

Fig. 1

2. Supporting infant's head and neck, turn on back and give four chest thrusts with 2-3 fingers 1/2" deep, at one finger-width below the nipples (mid-sternal region) *(Fig. 2)*

3. Repeat steps 1 and 2 until obstruction clears.

Fig. 2

> **Abdominal thrusts (Heimlich Maneuver) should not be done on an infant.**

Child (over 1 year) and adults

Ask "Are you choking?" If victim cannot speak, cough or breathe, take the following action (Heimlich Maneuver):

1. Kneel behind the child (stand behind a taller child or adult). *(Fig. 3)*

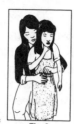

Fig. 3

2. Wrap your arms around the child's waist.

3. Make a fist with one hand. Place your fist (thumbside) against the child's stomach in the midline just above the navel and well below the rib cage.

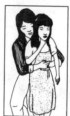

4. Grasp your fist with your other hand.

5. Press inward and upward into stomach with a quick thrust. *(Fig. 4)*

Fig. 4

6. Repeat thrust until obstruction is cleared.

> **Have someone call EMS # 911 immediately!**

> Do not give any form of nut, including peanuts or popcorn, hot dogs, hard candy, or whole grapes to children under five years old. These are common causes of choking in young children.

CHOKING (when child becomes unconscious)

Call EMS #911. If necessary, you can leave the phone off the hook and shout information into the phone while attending to the child.

Infant (birth to 1 year):

An infant who has become unconscious should be place in a supine (laying on back) position.

1. Perform jaw tongue lift *(Fig. 5)* and sweep the mouth only for visible objects. **Do not use "blind" finger sweeps** of the mouth as the object can be pushed back causing further obstruction.

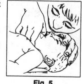

Fig. 5

2. Attempt to ventilate *(Fig. 6)*. If airway remains blocked proceed to step #3.

3. Perform 1 set of 4 back blows, then 4 chest thrusts (See Fig. 1 and 2).

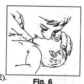

Fig. 6

Repeat steps 1, 2, and 3 until airway is clear or medical help arrives.

> **IMPORTANT:**
> If child is COUGHING - DO NOT INTERFERE!!!
> If child CANNOT COUGH, SPEAK or CRY, and/or is turning BLUE, use these techniques immediately!

Child (over 1 year) and adults

A child who has become unconscious should be placed in a supine (laying on back) position.

1. Perform jaw tongue lift *(Fig. 7)* and sweep the mouth only for visible objects. **Do not use "blind" finger sweeps** of the mouth on infants and children as the object can be pushed back causing further obstruction.

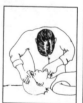

Fig. 7

2. Attempt to ventilate. If airway remains blocked proceed to step #3.

3. Deliver compressions by kneeling at the child's feet or straddling the child's legs, pressing the heel of one hand on the midline of the abdomen, slightly above the navel, pressing the free hand over the positioned hand and locking your elbows, and giving 6-10 rapid upward abdominal thrusts. *(Fig. 8)*

Fig. 8

Repeat steps 1, 2, & 3 until airway is clear.

Figures 5 and 6 reproduced with permission. Textbook of Pediatric Advanced Life Support, 1988, 1990 Copyright American Heart Association.

Source: *Childhood Emergencies—What to Do, A Quick Reference Guide,* by Marin Child Care Council (formerly Project Care for Children), Bull Publishing Company.

Constipation

Some people think that constipation means not having a bowel movement every day. Actually, the number of days between bowel movements isn't really the issue. Constipation is defined as having bowel movements that are hard and passed with pain or difficulty. An occasional hard stool need not cause special concern, but if a child has persistent constipation and her abdomen is swollen, her physician should examine her to make sure there isn't an underlying disease.

True constipation is rare in infants. There is a wide variation in the normal number of bowel movements a baby may have in a day, or even in a week; it isn't necessary to have one daily. It's also normal for infants to strain and turn red in the face while having a normal bowel movement, alarming as this may be to an adult bystander. Parents often change formulas hoping to solve this "problem," but generally it isn't necessary.

Toddlers sometimes develop constipation after they've had painful bowel movements. They hold them in, trying to avoid the discomfort. But what happens is that when they hold their bowel movements in, the intestines draw the water out of them, which makes them harder, which of course makes them hurt *worse.* You can see the potential for a vicious cycle here.

In these situations, physicians will often temporarily prescribe a stool softener. Hopefully, the child will get the idea that it doesn't always hurt to go to the bathroom, and he'll be more willing to "answer nature's call."

When older children are constipated, it is often because they can't use the bathroom when they need to, like when they're running on tight schedules or have to wait for recess at school. Also, some kids don't want to use school bathrooms, if they aren't given the privacy they want.

Maybe you're wondering at this point if we're ever going to talk about the role of nutrition in constipation. We're getting to that; but you should know that constipation can have other causes, too. So if you look at what a child's been eating, and there doesn't seem to be a problem with it, consider the factors mentioned above.[15]

Okay, now for the nutrition part. You are probably aware that fiber in foods contributes to regular bowel function. Fiber is the part of our food (usually plant matter) that we can't digest. It attracts water into the intestines, which makes the stool softer and bulkier. Most children don't get enough fiber in their diets. Most adults don't, either, actually.[15]

A daily diet that includes plenty of unprocessed foods and fresh produce will pretty much ensure adequate fiber intake. But you need to practice moderation in this regard. Children can end up deprived of needed nutrients when they're fanatically restricted to high-fiber, low-calorie foods. We generally don't recommend fiber supplements (like bran concentrates), either.

Constipation Prevention Plan

- Offer children fiber-rich foods often. Whole grains, fresh fruits and vegetables, dried fruits, dried beans, nuts, and popcorn are good sources of fiber.
- Make sure children drink water when they're thirsty. It helps fiber do its job.
- Encourage children to use the bathroom when they feel the urge to go, and allow them enough time to take care of their business. Make sure the bathroom is a pleasant enough place to be!
- Encourage plenty of physical activity. Exercise is thought to be beneficial in maintaining bowel regularity.

Dental Health

Nutrition affects the health of teeth in two ways. First, adequate amounts of certain nutrients are necessary for the formation of teeth. And secondly, the foods that go into the mouth can cause tooth decay.[16]

All of the primary ("baby") teeth and some of the permanent teeth are already forming in a baby's jaw before he is born. The teeth will depend upon proper nutrition for development until the last permanent tooth erupts. Sufficient amounts of *protein, calcium, phosphorus, magnesium, vitamin A, vitamin C, and vitamin D* must be present throughout this time if the teeth are to be well-formed. The minerals *fluoride, iron, and zinc* help make the teeth resistant to decay.

Most people don't realize that tooth decay is actually the result of an infection that is passed on to children by their parents or caregivers (babies aren't born with the bacteria that cause tooth decay in their mouths). We aren't telling you this to frighten you out of kissing your children! But the fact is that children tend to have fewer cavities when their parents practice good oral hygiene. So pay close attention . . . this is important for everybody.

The bacteria that cause tooth decay use the carbohydrates in the foods we eat, both for energy and for making substances that help them stick to the teeth in *plaque.* The bacteria also produce acids which dissolve the enamel of the teeth and form *cavities.*

You're probably already familiar with the sugars that feed these bacteria: table sugar, brown sugar, honey, maple syrup, molasses, and corn syrup are the principal ones. In addition, though, bacteria can get sugar by breaking down the starches in foods like potatoes and bread, if these foods stay in the mouth long enough.

You see, if a tooth is to end up with a cavity, three things are necessary:

- ❑ **bacteria** . . . to produce the acids that dissolve the tooth's enamel
- ❑ **carbohydrates** . . . to feed the bacteria and glue them to the tooth
- ❑ **time** . . . for the bacteria to do their work

When we talk about preventing cavities, we're generally trying to make sure at least one of the above factors is missing. For example, brushing teeth removes food particles, as well as some of the bacteria in the plaque.

---

20 Non-Candy Items That Children Love . . .
They will feel perfectly at home in
trick-or-treat bags, Christmas stockings, pinatas,
Easter baskets, or as party favors

- stickers
- pencils and pens
- erasers
- tiny farm animals
- pocket-size cars
- small books
- music tapes
- movie passes
- small bouncing balls
- jacks
- coins
- stamps for collecting
- colorful socks
- tangerines
- crayons
- little note pads
- individual packets of sunflower seeds or nuts
- dimestore jewelry
- hair ornaments

To Keep Tooth Decay Away[16]

❏ Serve a well-balanced diet, being careful to include good sources of calcium and phosphorus.

❏ Avoid foods that are high in sugar, like soda pop, candy, cookies, pastries, jams, syrups, and presweetened breakfast cereals.

❏ Avoid foods that stick to the teeth. Raisins, other dried fruits, fruit rolls, and gummy-style fruit candies fall into this category.

❏ Serve raw vegetables often. They scrub the teeth and stimulate the flow of saliva, which can help protect the teeth.

❏ If you are going to serve a sweet food, do it at mealtime, not as an ongoing snack. This will cut down on the amount of time the teeth are exposed to the sugar.

❏ Encourage children to brush their teeth after meals. If that's not possible, they should at least floss and brush their teeth once a day. Be sure children brush their teeth after eating sticky foods.

❏ Children should be drinking fluoridated water. Find out whether your water supply has fluoride. Bottled waters have differing levels, too.

❏ *Never send a child to bed with a bottle, unless it has plain water in it.*

❏ ❏ ❏

Diabetes and Other Chronic Diseases

The purpose of this section is not to give you specific instructions about caring for children with diabetes or other diseases. Rather, we're going to bring up some of the issues related to nutrition that frequently arise in these circumstances, and we'll pass on some suggestions for handling them.

Parents and caregivers are usually very concerned about doing the right thing for a child with a chronic health condition, as they should be. But things go better when they are neither intimidated nor overprotective. It's important to follow the medical treatment plan, but at the same time to allow the child to take increasing responsibility for himself, with the chance to enjoy being as much like other children as possible.

While the health conditions we will describe are quite different, there are common nutritional issues that are bound to come up when you are caring for children who have any one of them:

❏ It can be difficult to follow the prescribed dietary plan without interfering with a child's decisions about the kinds and amounts of foods to eat.[20]

❏ Children generally detest being treated differently from other children, and they will probably resent having to eat special foods.

❏ Children with chronic diseases need to learn self-care skills; this includes making appropriate food choices in unsupervised situations.

❏ These children may use the tactic of eating forbidden foods, or not eating at all, to manipulate their parents' and caregivers' behavior.

Diabetes

About one in every 600 children develops diabetes, usually the "insulin dependent" form of the disease. The bodies of most people produce the hormone insulin, which moves glucose (sugar) from the blood into the cells of the body, where it can be used for energy. People with diabetes either don't produce insulin, or what insulin they have isn't effective. So the glucose ends up hanging around in the bloodstream, while the cells are starving for their fuel. High blood sugars can have serious short-term and long-term consequences.[17]

Treatment of "insulin dependent" diabetes generally involves (1) injections of insulin to make up for what's lacking in the body, (2) a food plan formulated to avoid very high or very low blood sugars, and to provide the nutrients for normal growth and development, and (3) a program of exercise, which helps stabilize blood sugars and maintain normal weight.

In order to care for a child with diabetes, you will need to know:[17]

- ❑ the symptoms of *hypoglycemia* (low blood sugar) and *ketoacidosis* (the result of high blood sugars), and what to do about them

- ❑ how to plan meals and snacks; you will need to consider the types of food offered, the amounts, and the timing. The diabetic diet is basically the same healthy diet we recommend for everyone!

- ❑ when necessary, how to help the child test blood sugars and inject insulin

- ❑ how to help the child manage her exercise regime

Cystic Fibrosis

Cystic fibrosis is an inherited glandular disease. It affects digestion and absorption, causes the loss of vital minerals in the sweat, and can lead to chronic lung infections. Treatment may include pancreatic enzyme replacement for better digestion and antibiotics to fight off infections.

Children with cystic fibrosis often don't get the nourishment from their food needed to help them grow well. It can be a real challenge to help them meet their need for extra calories. They may require specially formulated fats that they can absorb better, extra salt when they've been sweating a lot, and certain vitamin and mineral supplements.[18]

Inborn Errors of Metabolism

Some children are born without the enzymes necessary to handle particular food elements such as sugars or amino acids. Toxic levels of these elements can build up in the blood, causing damage to the nervous system and hindering growth. Phenylketonuria (PKU), galactosemia, and fructose intolerance are examples of inborn errors of metabolism that call for strict dietary modifications. Often special formulas and food products are necessary.[19]

❑ ❑ ❑

Diarrhea

Diarrhea has been defined as the passage of frequent, watery stools. There are some children who have bowel movements that are normal for them but look like diarrhea, just as some children have bowel movements so infrequently that their parents think they're constipated. Parents and caregivers have to determine what is normal for a particular child.[21] In addition to being a bother, to say the least, diarrhea can have an effect on a child's nutritional status. And what a child is eating can sometimes be a cause of diarrhea.

Acute Diarrhea

Acute diarrhea is usually caused by a viral or bacterial infection (called "enteritis"), and may be accompanied by a fever and vomiting. It can be a serious problem for infants or very young children because they can become dehydrated quite easily.

Consequently, many parents are now using glucose-electrolyte maintenance beverages like Pedialyte® or Ricelyte® to replace fluids lost from vomiting, diarrhea, and fever. These beverages are readily available in supermarkets and drug stores, but they should only be used as advised by a physician. *They are not meant to be used as substitutes for feeding.* Parents and caregivers often make the mistake of waiting too long to resume feeding a child who has had a bout with enteritis. While eating *will* cause more stool volume, the child actually does gain some value from the food.

Here's what the American Academy of Pediatrics recommends:[22]

❑ Don't feed the child if he is vomiting a lot, has significant dehydration, or his abdomen is swollen (call the doctor!).

❑ When there is no vomiting or dehydration, resume feeding the child:
  • Infants can usually tolerate breast milk well.
  • Some infants need to drink lactose-free formula for a few days, but many will do fine when their regular formula is merely diluted at first.

- Older children should be offered carbohydrate-rich foods like bananas, potatoes, and rice cereal.
- Within a few days the child should be eating normally.

Chronic Nonspecific Diarrhea

Also called "toddler diarrhea," this condition can occur any time between six months and 4 1/2 years of age. The child will have four or five stools a day, four or five days out of a month, yet have no specific diseases and exhibit normal growth and development.[23] Chronic nonspecific diarrhea isn't particularly dangerous, but it is messy, and in some cases dietary changes can help solve the problem. It may be worth experimenting a bit with diet rather than just waiting for the child to outgrow the condition.

- ❑ Susceptible children can get diarrhea when fat is restricted too severely in their diets. Fat slows down the digestive process, so adding some fat to the diets of these children may alleviate the diarrhea.[24]

- ❑ Children may also develop diarrhea when they're allowed to drink excessive amounts of juice or sweetened liquids. Some children seem to have a sensitivity to the sugars in juices and will get diarrhea when they drink even modest amounts.[25,26,27]

- ❑ It's a good idea to avoid serving foods with artificial sweeteners to children, as these may contribute to diarrhea.[21]

- ❑ It is usually *not* necessary to restrict dairy products, eggs, or wheat in the diets of children with chronic diarrhea, and in fact children are at risk of nutrient deficiencies when such restrictions are applied without careful planning.[28]

Eating Disorders

Lots of parents consider their children to be problem eaters. It's normal for children to go through periods of lagging appetites, pickiness, and preferring candy bars to vegetables. But occasionally a child's eating problem is serious enough to be called an *eating disorder.* It may manifest itself as failure to thrive, obesity, excessive pickiness, or monumental struggles between the child and the parent or caregiver about eating. (What we usually think of as eating disorders—anorexia nervosa and bulimia—don't show up until adolescence or later.)

Child feeding expert Ellyn Satter stresses that an eating disorder consists of a severe disturbance in eating or feeding accompanied by an emotional problem. There are lots of circumstances in which eating disorders can develop, from parental pressure to eat more or less food, to problems in their marital relationship. When the adults are trying to exercise an inappropriate amount of control over a child's eating, when the situation is very charged emotionally, and when no one is willing to change, it's time to see a therapist. The underlying emotional issues need to be resolved before eating can return to normal.[29]

Helping to Prevent Eating Disorders

- It's important for a family to be functioning well and for the individual family members to be emotionally healthy.
- Adults should be role models for healthy attitudes toward eating and body image.
- The child should be supported in following his own internal sense of food regulation. Parents and caregivers should neither withhold food from a child nor force a child to eat.
- Teach the child to feel good about herself, no matter what body size and shape she has acquired.

❑ ❑ ❑

Food-Drug Interactions

Rare is the child who at some time doesn't receive medication for an illness. She may need to take antibiotics for a short time when she has an infection, or she may require long-term drug therapy for asthma or seizures. Many people are unaware that foods and medications can interact with each other to produce some unwanted effects. This is important to know when dealing with children, because they may suffer longer from their illnesses or experience poor growth and nutrient deficiencies if the food-drug interactions aren't taken into account.

Foods can alter the effectiveness of a drug by:
- ❑ either reducing or increasing the amount of the drug absorbed
- ❑ changing the way the drug is used in the body
- ❑ causing more or less of the drug to be excreted in the urine

Drugs can affect a child's nutritional state by:
- ❑ changing the way foods taste and smell
- ❑ increasing or reducing appetite
- ❑ causing nausea, vomiting, or diarrhea
- ❑ changing the amounts of nutrients that are absorbed
- ❑ altering the way nutrients are used in the body
- ❑ causing more or less of a nutrient to be excreted in the urine[31]

When You Must Administer Medications to a Child, Ask, Among Other Things:

- whether the drug should be taken with food or on an empty stomach
- if there are any foods which should be *avoided*
- if any nutrients should be *emphasized*

Call a pharmacist if you have any questions about food-drug interactions

---

❑ ❑ ❑

"Junk Food"

We resist labeling foods as "good" or "bad"; rather, we think that there are "good eating habits" and "bad eating habits." "Good eating habits" provide the necessary nutrients in appropriate amounts to maintain well-being. "Bad eating habits" do not.

It's hard to think of any foods that would actually be harmful for most children to eat *once in a while.* But it's easy to name dozens of foods that have very little nutritional value and could lead to health problems if consumed *frequently.* These are what concerned adults call "junk foods," and they are characteristically high in sugar, salt, or fat. Candy, cookies, sodas, and snack chips are examples.

Parents and caregivers have valid concerns about children eating these foods:

- ❑ Frequent consumption of sugary foods can cause tooth decay.
- ❑ Eating a lot of "junk foods" can give a child less appetite for the truly nutritious foods he needs for growth.
- ❑ It's easy to take in too many calories when eating foods high in fat and sugar (however, research has not shown that overweight children eat any more high-calorie foods than thinner children do).[32]

The problem is, children don't look at the situation this way. Remember what we said early in this book about the reasons people eat as they do (page 8)? Well, children aren't particularly worried about developing nutrient deficiencies; they just know they like to eat foods that taste good to them.

The sweetness or saltiness of "junk foods" makes them particularly attractive to children (and adults). Babies are *born* with a preference for sweet flavors, and children can acquire a taste for salt, even cravings for it, when they've habitually eaten salty foods.[33] Children also want to eat what they just *know* other kids are eating.

Adults and children can get into some major battles over "junk foods." Parents and caregivers who are sincerely trying to provide good nutrition for kids may prohibit them from eating these foods. What usually happens next isn't too surprising when you consider human nature; the foods that are forbidden become *very* attractive to these children. Have you ever noticed the way children whose parents "never" allow them to eat foods with sugar go absolutely wild over sweets at parties and grandparents' houses?

Yes, it's true that we don't *need* junk foods. Most of us are better off without them, especially as we grow older and more sedentary, and our caloric needs go down. But since it is unlikely that sweet, fatty, and salty foods are going to disappear anytime soon, and since many people find them enjoyable, the reasonable thing to do is teach children how to work them into an otherwise healthful way of eating.

As we said earlier, eating a piece of candy every now and then is unlikely to do any harm; it's when candy is providing a significant portion of a child's calories that nutritional problems will occur. You can maintain your commitment to good nutrition and allow children to experience an occasional cupcake or handful of snack chips.

❑ The best way to teach children how to manage "junk foods" is to serve them occasionally without any more fuss than you would for carrot sticks or cheese slices. If the children ask why they can't have these foods more often, just let them know that they aren't as good for them as other foods, but they're okay once in a while.[34]

❑ Minimize the damage by making your own nutritious versions of junk foods. You can make cookies with less sugar, muffins instead of frosted cupcakes, or baked potato sticks rather than french fries.

❑ Emphasize the other celebratory aspects of holidays and birthdays besides eating. Plan lots of games, songs, storytelling, and similar activities. Give prizes and party favors that aren't candy (see page 196).

❑ *Never* use foods as rewards for good behavior or as consolation for upsets and injuries.

❑ Be careful about the amount of time children spend watching television. It's hard for kids not to be interested in nutritionally questionable foods when confronted with such dazzling advertising for them.

❑   ❑   ❑

Lactose Intolerance

Lactose is a form of sugar that is found in almost all animal milks, including human milk. If a person doesn't have the enzymes in the small intestine to digest lactose (which is the case for *most* adults in the world), it goes into the large intestine where bacteria ferment the stuff. This fermentation process results in acids and gases that can cause abdominal cramps, flatulence, and diarrhea.[35]

Children can generally handle the lactose in dairy products until they're about five or six years old. After that, their tolerance to lactose will depend upon their heredity. (Scientists tell us that Northern Europeans, Hungarians, members of the Fulani and Tussi tribes in Africa, the Punjabi from India, and perhaps Mongolians are able to digest lactose as adults. The rest of the world's peoples cannot, unless they can count some of these "lactose digesters" among their ancestors).[35]

A physician can determine whether a child is lactose intolerant by administering some special tests. If it turns out that a child does have this problem, you will need to make some changes in what you're feeding him:

❑ Many people with lactose intolerance can digest fermented dairy dairy products: yogurt, hard cheese, cottage cheese, and acidophilus milk.

❑ Enzyme preparations, such as Lactaid®, can be added to milk; they "predigest" the lactose.

❑ Some children can tolerate regular milk if they simply drink smaller portions of it, more frequently.

❑ If a child is unable to tolerate *any* dairy products, be sure to offer him foods rich in the nutrients he'll be missing, like calcium.

❑   ❑   ❑

Low-Fat Diets and Children

Several health organizations have made dietary recommendations aimed at reducing our risks of heart disease, cancer, and stroke. Common to all of them is the advice to limit fat intake to no more than 30% of calories, to cut the saturated fat in our diets to 10% of calories or less, and to eat less cholesterol.[36] Many adults are taking these recommendations seriously, eating less red meat, taking the skin off their chicken, and switching from whole milk to low-fat or non-fat milk. And they're wondering if it's OK to do the same for their children.

Actually, health experts disagree, sometimes quite heatedly, on the matter. The two big questions that need to be settled are: Does what children eat affect their chance of getting chronic diseases like atherosclerosis when they're adults? And will restricting the fat in their diets lead to poor growth or nutrient deficiencies?

There's been a lot of research looking at the relationship between lifestyle factors (including diet) and heart disease. Some of the findings have led experts to recommend low-fat diets for children:[37]

❑ In countries where adults have high rates of heart disease, both children and adults have higher blood cholesterol levels than in countries where the incidence of heart disease is low.

❑ People from countries where heart disease rates and blood cholesterol levels are lower tend to eat less saturated fat and cholesterol than people from countries with higher heart disease rates.

❑ Children develop fatty streaks in their blood vessels, which may develop into the lesions of atherosclerosis at an early age.

Not everyone is convinced that low-fat diets for children are necessary or safe, however. The American Academy of Pediatrics has taken a cautious view, stating that the evidence that a low-fat diet in childhood will prevent heart disease is not strong enough. The Academy also expresses concern that children won't receive enough calories for growth or important nutrients like iron and calcium when red meats or dairy products are restricted in their diets.[37]

In some cases, these fears have been justified. There have been reports of children who suffered growth failure because their parents limited the fats in their diets too strictly.[38,39] But other researchers have found that when parents get the right supervision from health professionals, children on low-fat diets can grow just fine.[40]

No doubt the controversy will rage on for years. Meanwhile, perhaps the best argument for providing low-fat foods to children is that their eating patterns are formed in childhood. It isn't necessary to count every gram of fat a child takes in; what's important is that he learns while he's young to enjoy eating poultry, seafood, low-fat dairy products, whole grains, fruits, and vegetables. It will be much harder to change his eating habits when he's an adult.

It appears that low-fat diets are safe, and probably beneficial, for most children.[36] Earlier in this book you found suggestions for reducing fat in the foods you serve (pages 64–66). Keep in mind that there are other risk factors for heart disease that are important to work on during childhood and adolescence, such as obesity, lack of physical fitness, and cigarette smoking.[37]

- ❑ *Never* restrict fat in the diet of a child less than two years old.

- ❑ Don't restrict fat in the diet of a child who is underweight and a fussy eater.

- ❑ Avoid getting too involved in what children are eating. Offer healthful choices, but don't hover over them, monitoring every pat of butter or slice of cheese.

- ❑ Children may need to eat more often, because foods low in fat aren't satisfying for long, and because they may not be able to eat enough at the usual meals to get the calories they require.

- ❑ Be a good role model for a healthy lifestyle, conscientious without being fanatic. You've heard the old saying . . . too much worrying about your health can be bad for your health!

❑ ❑ ❑

Overweight Children

Our society has an obsession with thinness. And in the midst of this obsession, more and more children are becoming overweight, or to be more precise, obese. (Obesity is excessive body fat, versus overweight, in which the excessive weight could be coming from heavy bones, large muscles, or too much fat. We will use the terms somewhat interchangeably, because heavy children have certain problems regardless of where their weight comes from). A recent report stated that 29% of 6- to 11-year-old boys and 26% of girls the same age in the United States are obese.[41]

Heavy children are likely to be viewed as unlikeable or lacking in self-control. They may suffer a poor self-image and sense of failure, and they will undoubtably feel pressure to lose weight by dieting. Whether these children will be obese as adults will relate to how long they've been obese, how obese they are, and whether or not they are obese as adolescents.

Adult health problems associated with obesity include high blood pressure, respiratory diseases, gallstones, orthopedic conditions, and diabetes. During childhood, it's generally believed that obesity causes more social and psychological problems than physical ones.[42]

Why are some people obese? The basic reason is that they have taken in more calories than their bodies can use, so the leftovers are stored as fat. But contrary to popular belief, obese people don't necessarily eat more than thinner ones. There seem to be many reasons why some people gain excess fat and others don't:[43]

- ❏ heredity
- ❏ lack of physical activity
- ❏ the composition of the diet (calories from fat appear to be stored as fat more easily than calories from other sources)[44]
- ❏ slower metabolism, which is largely inborn but may be influenced by such factors as repeated attempts at weight loss or the number of daily meals
- ❏ overeating, which may be the result of:[42]
  - • eating too fast
  - • being out of touch with true feelings of hunger and satisfaction
  - • eating in response to stress or traumatic events

Unfortunately, well-meaning adults sometimes use tactics with overweight children that cause more serious problems than the overweight itself. Putting pressure on children about their weight can lead to:[45]

- ❏ obsessions about food, dieting, and body image
- ❏ lowered self-esteem and an overwhelming sense of failure on the child's part
- ❏ damage to the adult-child relationship in the midst of battles over food choices, food quantities, and exercise

The most common mistake that parents and some physicians make is putting children on diets or being overly restrictive with their eating. For one thing, as mentioned earlier, not all overweight children are big eaters. Limiting their calories may interfere with normal growth and development. Furthermore, children who aren't allowed to eat until they feel satisfied may feel deprived and singled out, and they tend to become obsessed with eating. And when adults exert too much control over what children eat, the children never learn to manage eating for themselves.[45]

Overweight children are victims of other strong-arm tactics, as well. One mother told us of the humiliation her daughter felt when her upper-arm fatfold measurements were read aloud to her sixth-grade class. And this very conscientious young student received a failing grade in her gym class because she couldn't quite run a mile. Can you imagine how this girl might feel about her body and exercise when she grows up . . . thanks to these early experiences?

We aren't advocating letting overweight children (or any children, for that matter) eat whatever they want, whenever they want. And we don't think children should be encouraged to spend all of their free time curled up in front of the television set, either. Adults are *supposed* to be in charge of the kinds of foods that are offered to children and the timing of meals and snacks.[45] And adults *should* be setting limits on sedentary activities like watching television.

But all of this can be done in ways that leave a child's self-esteem intact and teach him to make his own lifestyle decisions. We also need to recognize that we don't *know* how a child's body will turn out when she's older, nor do we need to subscribe to society's rather limited view of what constitutes the "ideal body."

❑   ❑   ❑

Pesticides and Other Chemicals in Our Food

Consumers are told that the American food supply is the "safest in the world," yet many grow increasingly uncomfortable with the idea of "all those chemicals in our food." Some of these fears seem to be justified, and others are not. After all, even "natural" foods are made up of chemicals; for that matter, so are our bodies.

Not all "natural" chemicals are good for us, just as not all synthetic chemicals are bad. Most of us can accept that. What we resent is that invisible substances which could cause cancer, birth defects, or other problems may be lurking in our food without there being good reasons for them being there!

Much of the recent furor over contaminants in foods has involved pesticide residues. The "Alar scare" in 1989 brought the issue of pesticide residues in foods to our attention in a big way. Parents, especially, were concerned about the dangers their children might face while eating the very fruits and vegetables that were supposed to be *good* for them. Meanwhile respected scientists debated the hazards and virtues of pesticides, as they probably will continue to do for many years. To stimulate your thinking (and inquiring), we will summarize the points of controversy for you.

Experts who feel that pesticide residues in our foods are of grave danger to our health assert that:[46,47]

❑   Many of the ingredients in pesticides have not been tested thoroughly for their toxic effects.

❑   The Food and Drug Administration has only established tolerated amounts or "action levels" for a fraction of the chemicals in our food.

❑   Action levels are set with the assumption that a consumer eats a certain amount of a food (for example, one avocado, 1 1/2 cups of cooked summer squash, or 2 1/2 tangerines per year)

❏ Many pesticides aren't detected by the tests now in use.

❏ Imported foods may contain residues of pesticides that are banned in the United States.

❏ Children face greater risks from pesticides because:

- They eat more for their body weight of the foods likely to have high levels of contaminants (they eat more fruit and drink more apple juice, for example).

- They're more susceptible to the effects of toxins and cancer-causing substances, because their body cells are dividing rapidly, and their immune systems are immature.

- They will be living longer than people who are adults now, so cancer will have a longer time to show up in their bodies.

There are scientists who feel that the risks from pesticides are exaggerated. They argue that:[48]

❏ We eat a lot more natural pesticides, those which are made by plants in self-defense, than synthetic ones, and at least half of these natural compounds may be able to cause cancer.

❏ We have general bodily defenses against **all** toxins, no matter what their source.

❏ Many fruits and vegetables contain substances that probably prevent cancer, and the benefits from these foods outweigh the risks.

❏ Consumers may not be able to afford enough fruits and vegetables if the more "natural" methods increase their cost.

While health experts disagree on the extent of the hazards posed by pesticide residues, they do agree that it's better to go ahead and eat fruits and vegetables than to avoid them out of fear. There **are** steps you can take to minimize your exposure to pesticides. We'll outline them for you at the end of this section.

Food (and water) may contain other contaminants as well. Fungal poisons, heavy metals like lead and mercury, industrial chemicals, animal hormones and antibiotic residues, chemicals that migrate into food from packaging, and food colorings, flavorings, and many other food additives have the potential to cause health problems. Some of this contamination occurs naturally; some is the outcome of poorly-handled industrial waste, agricultural practices, and consumer demand for foods that taste and look a certain way. Changes will be needed in industrial practices and governmental enforcement to solve some of these problems.

You don't have to feel like a victim, however; you can do a lot to make sure the foods you serve are as safe as possible. For one thing, realize that one of the greatest dangers we face is food poisoning from bacteria or viruses . . . a product of our *own* mishandling of food.

Serve a wide variety of foods and "spread out" the potential contaminants. Seek out foods that are organically grown or free of artificial colorings and flavorings. Remember, you "vote" with your shopping dollars! Know where your food comes from; avoid, for example, buying fish caught in polluted waters. And you can keep yourself informed about these issues by subscribing to such publications as the *Nutrition Action Healthletter* or writing to:

Americans for Safe Food
1501 16th St., NW
Washington, DC 20036

How to Minimize Your Exposure to Pesticides[46]

❏ Buy produce that is grown organically or with Integrated Pest Management.

❏ Buy produce that has been grown in the United States, especially broccoli, bell peppers, melons, cauliflower, green beans, tomatoes, and cucumbers. The produce manager at your market should be able to tell you where such items were grown.

❏ Wash fruits and vegetables in water to which you've added a few drops of dishwashing detergent; use a scrub brush and rinse well.

❏ Peel produce that has been waxed; it's obvious when cucumbers have been waxed, but apples, bell peppers, citrus fruits, eggplants, tomatoes, sweet potatoes, and squash may be waxed as well. Stores *should* have a sign letting consumers know when produce has been waxed.

❏ Trim the fat from meat, poultry, and fish. These foods, as well as butter and lard, may contain *more* pesticide residues than produce! That's because pesticides tend to accumulate in fat.

❏ Peas and dried beans usually have the lowest levels of pesticide residues . . . serve them often! Besides, they're very nutritious and inexpensive.

❏ Plant a garden and grow your own. Better yet, let the children do it.

❏ ❏ ❏

Sodium

Sodium is an essential mineral for the functioning of our bodies. However, the amount we need is actually *very* small compared to the amount many of us consume.

The sodium in our food is primarily in the form of *sodium chloride,* or table salt; a teaspoon of salt contains about 2,000 milligrams of sodium. Some sodium is also contributed by additives like sodium bicarbonate (baking soda) and monosodium glutamate (MSG). Only about 10% of the sodium in our foods is naturally present; the rest is added during cooking and at the table (15%) and during food manufacturing (75%). Cereals and baked goods, processed meats, and dairy products are the major sources of sodium in the American diet.[49]

Many consumers have been trying to cut down on salt consumption because of evidence that connects sodium with high blood pressure. Actually, most people don't develop high blood pressure from eating a lot of salt. But it's impossible to predict who will and who won't, so health authorities recommend moderation in sodium intake for everybody.

No one has been able to prove that children can get high blood pressure from eating a lot of salt,[36] but it is clear that a preference for salty foods can be cultivated by eating them frequently.[33] This could lead to problems later on, if these children grow up to be some of the adults who do develop hypertension as the result of salt sensitivity.

It makes sense, then, to exercise moderation in your use of salt and foods high in sodium when feeding children. They should learn to enjoy the natural taste of foods. Suggestions for reducing salt during your food preparation are on page 68.

While they have not issued specific guidelines for children's sodium intake, health experts are advising that we all keep our daily sodium intake below about 2,500 milligrams.[36]

Sodium in Foods Children Commonly Eat*

Food	Milligrams of Sodium
Corn flake cereal (1 oz)	351
Shredded wheat biscuits (1 oz)	3
Tomato soup (10 oz)	1,050
Tomato juice (8 oz)	744
Milk (8 oz)	130
Orange juice (8 oz)	2
Lowfat cottage cheese (1/2 c)	435
Processed American cheese (1 oz)	238
Cheddar cheese (1 oz)	190
Plain lowfat yogurt (1 c)	159
Beef hot dog (1)	425
Bologna (2 slices)	450
Tuna, water-packed (2 oz)	312
Chicken breast, roasted (2 oz)	42
Peanut butter (2 T)	167
Canned baked beans (1 c)	810
Canned spaghetti and meatballs (7.5 oz)	1,000
Pizza (1 slice)	500–1,000
Fast-food deluxe hamburger	1,510
Cheese goldfish crackers (10)	117
Pretzel (1)	54
Butter-flavor crackers (3)	97
Tortilla chips (1 oz)	99
Dill pickle (2 oz)	700
Mustard (1 T)	212
Ketchup (1 T)	154
Mayonnaise (1 T)	80

❏   ❏   ❏

Special Needs and Feeding

Children with developmental or physical disabilities are prone to the same nutritional problems that affect their peers: obesity, iron-deficiency anemia, underweight, and tooth decay. Their risks of nutritient deficiencies and excesses are greater, however, because they may have trouble eating, or have altered nutrient requirements. And it can be more difficult for a child with disabilities to develop the self-esteem that comes, among other things, from successfully managing eating.

*Sources: *Sodium Scoreboard*. Center for Science in the Public Interest, 1501 16th St, NW, Washington, DC 20036.
Wrap-up: sodium. *University of California, Berkeley, Wellness Letter* 2(7): 4, 1986.

Nutrition-related concerns that may arise when a child has developmental delays or physical handicaps include:

❑ an increased requirement for calories, due to medications, diseases, or central nervous system damage

❑ a reduced requirement for calories, due to inactivity, slow metabolism, or medications; this can lead to obesity

❑ drug-nutrient interactions, which may change vitamin needs

❑ lack of sensation of hunger or satiety in some children with central nervous system damage

❑ feeding difficulties:

  • limited sucking ability (infants)

  • inability to sit up and balance the head

  • lack of strength or control in the arms and wrists

  • difficulty coordinating biting, chewing, and swallowing without choking or drooling

  • difficulty grasping utensils or removing food from them

  • excessive gagging and vomiting

  • extreme sensitivity to food temperatures

❑ constipation, resulting from slowed bowel action, inactivity, lack of fiber in the diet, or inadequate fluids[52]

It can be quite a challenge to manage your feeding relationship with a child who has a disability. She will go through the same developmental sequence of eating skills and behaviors that you would expect of any child, but she will probably do it more slowly. It may be very tempting to feed her only the foods that she can eat very easily, or not to let her feed herself because she makes such a mess. It might also be tempting to try to make her eat more or eat less when you are concerned about how she's growing.

Children with handicaps are entitled to, and need, the benefits of good nutrition as much as any other children. They are also entitled to progress as far as possible in their development, to have as much control over their lives as they can, and to be treated respectfully, with consideration for their feelings and comfort.[52] It is outside of the scope of this book to teach you the specifics of feeding children with special needs, but we will give you some general guidelines:

❑ Allow the child to eat foods of progressively more challenging textures as he appears able.

  • Avoid prolonged use of bottle-feeding.

  • Be alert for cues (they may be subtle) that the child is ready for solid foods and coarser textures.

❑ Help the child to develop self-feeding skills.

  • Don't feed a child if he is at all capable of feeding himself.

  • Make sure the child is comfortable; supports for his head, arms, trunk, or feet may be necessary so that he can sit upright.

  • He may need adaptive feeding equipment.

  • Take it step by step, allowing the child to experience success before moving on to more difficult skills.

❑ Respect the child's preferences regarding types and amounts of food eaten (from what *you* offer, of course), pace of eating, and even whether he will eat.

❑ Avoid overindulgence with sweet foods and unlimited snacking. Children with handicaps need limits, too.

❑ Find out if any of the child's medications interact with nutrients.

❑ When you would like training or you're having problems feeding a child with special needs, seek out professionals in your community who can help: occupational therapists, physical therapists, speech therapists, dietitians, and behavior modification specialists. See *Appendix D—Resources* for more information.

❑   ❑   ❑

Sugar, Food Additives, and Children's Behavior

Parents exchange knowing looks when a mother describes how her darling child turned into a monster during the days following Halloween. And teachers fear that birthday-party cupcakes will send an entire class into a hyperkinetic frenzy. Actually, all kids get "wild" sometimes.

Between one and five percent of children develop *hyperkinesis,* also known as attention deficit disorder or hyperactivity. This disorder is characterized by overactivity, distractibility, impulsive behavior, and a low tolerance for frustration. No one really knows what causes it.[7] But desperate, exhausted parents sometimes wonder if there might be something to all this talk about sugar and food additives, especially food colorings.

Despite the popularity of the Feingold diet in the 1970s, it has been very hard for scientists to prove that there is a link between dietary components and hyperactivity. When a child's diet is changed, his behavior may improve because his parents expect it to. Or there might be changes in family dynamics. Maybe the child feels better because he's eating a more nourishing diet than he was before.

Generally, research trials in which neither the parents, the child, nor the observers knew whether the child received sugar (or an additive) or a placebo have failed to find a connection between dietary components and behavior.[7,53] Some studies have even indicated that sugar has a calming effect on children.[54]

Most health experts believe that there are other reasons why children get "hyper" after they've eaten sugar, such as the general excitement or fatigue that accompanies celebrations. Maybe they become super-excited about being able to indulge in otherwise "forbidden" treats. However, we must say that some research studies have found that a very small number of children *do* respond to sugar or additives with behavior changes.[7,55] The results of a recent study, albeit a small one, suggest that children's hormones may respond differently from adults', to large doses of sugar.[56]

It's a good idea to consult a physician before imposing an unnecessarily restrictive diet on a child. Diets completely free of sugar and food additives can be a lot of work for the adults and traumatic for the child.

At the same time, there are good reasons for limiting the amounts of sugar and additives in the foods you serve. Sugar causes tooth decay. Eating lots of sugary foods can displace other more nutritious foods in the diet, leading to borderline nutrition. And while some food additives seem to be safe, there are questions about the safety of others, including some coloring agents, nitrates, nitrites, and saccharin. Many additives, especially colorings, can be easily avoided.

There are other aspects of children's food patterns that can have effects on their behavior. They are:[53]

Nutrient deficiencies   Deficiencies of most nutrients will affect behavior. The most common deficiency in the United States is iron deficiency. The brain is very sensitive to a lack of iron, and this can have profound effects: fatigue, distractibility, irritability, reduced tolerance for challenging tasks, and headaches.

Skipping meals   Children need to eat every 4 to 6 hours to supply their brains with needed glucose. Children who skip breakfast or other meals tend to be irritable and unable to concentrate on the tasks at hand. That's why midmorning snacks are a good idea, and why kids should eat their breakfast!

Caffeine   This is often overlooked as a source of "wild" behavior in children. But for a child's size, a 12-ounce can of cola contains the caffeine equivalent to 3 or 4 cups of coffee for an adult.

Food allergies   While most allergists don't believe that food allergies themselves can cause behavior problems, a child who feels miserable because of allergy symptoms is likely to be difficult to manage.

This sounds like the same old-fashioned advice we heard when we were children, but there really is no substitute for regular, well-balanced meals and snacks, regular sleep, and regular exercise. It's a good idea to monitor television viewing, too; many of the shows children like are violent and overstimulating. Sometimes the simplest interventions are the last ones we consider. Consider them first!

❏   ❏   ❏

Television

The average child in the United States spends more time watching televison than in any other activity except sleeping. It is estimated that 2- to 5 year-olds watch 25 hours of televison per week, children aged 6 to 11 watch 22 hours per week, and adolescents watch 23 hours per week. How all of this television viewing affects a child will depend upon how long she does it and what she sees while she does it.[57] Television can have a *considerable* impact on children's nutrition, as you will see.

Here's what nutritionists don't like about television:[58]

❏ It's a sedentary activity.

❏ Children see about 20,000 commercials a year,[59] of which about half promote foods of low nutritional value.[60] Younger children are particularly inclined to believe claims that the products being advertised are *good* for them.

❏ It encourages children to manipulate their parents' purchasing decisions at the grocery store.

- ❏ It is conducive to mindless snacking.
- ❏ It can hinder social interaction at mealtimes.
- ❏ It promotes obesity[41] and high blood cholesterol levels.[61]

Television does have its good features, however:[58]

- ❏ It can be a source of useful information presented in a way that is very attractive to children.
- ❏ It can be a trigger for talking about nutrition and health behaviors.

Watching television may not be an option in your home or child care center. If it is, there are ways you can emphasize its positive aspects and downplay the negative.

Television and Good Nutrition
***Can* Be Friends**

- Be selective about what children are watching. Some stations make more of an effort to present nutrition friendly messages than others.
- Watch television *with* the children. Talk about the eating and health behaviors portrayed on the programs. Discuss the ways consumers can be misled by advertising.
- Limit viewing time. Balance passive activities like television watching with physical activity.
- *Don't allow children to eat while they watch television.*

❏ ❏ ❏

Underweight Children

Some children are destined to be small. Others have the potential to grow larger or more quickly, but for some reason they don't. Sometimes in our weight-conscious society we get very concerned about a child who is overweight, yet fail to notice when a child isn't growing as well as she could. But faltering growth can be a serious problem, with many causes:[62]

- ❏ Some children require more calories for their size than others, due to heredity or activity, and caregivers may underestimate their food needs.
- ❏ Children may eat poorly because they are exceedingly finicky, can't handle sitting at the table for long, are resistant to what they perceive as pressure to eat, or suffer from anxiety or depression.
- ❏ Children have grown poorly when their parents severely restricted fat or calories in their diets.

- Children may have limited self-feeding skills or difficulty chewing and swallowing the food that is offered.
- Certain disease processes can interfere with growth.

A child who is lagging in her growth should be evaluated by a physician, of course, and treatments vary. But you as a parent or caregiver can do much to help the underweight child by:[62]

- making sure that you provide a supportive and attractive environment for eating
- providing regular meals and snacks, including foods the child enjoys, with *no pressure* on the child to eat
- checking to make sure there's enough fat in the child's diet
- observing whether the child has any problems with chewing or swallowing the foods you offer; you may be offering foods too advanced for the child, or she may need professional help.
- being alert to signs that the child is anxious, withdrawn, or depressed; therapy may be in order
- accepting the child's body, no matter how she turns out

❑ ❑ ❑

Vegetarianism

People may choose not to eat meat, or any foods of animal origin, for religious, health, ethical, or political reasons. Much of the world's population is vegetarian because they can't afford meat. Some vegetarians eat no meat, poultry, or fish but do eat eggs and dairy products (*lacto-ovo-vegetarians*), some avoid eggs as well (*lacto-vegetarians*), and some eat no animal products whatsoever (*vegans*).

The vegetarian diet can't guarantee good health, just as eating meat doesn't guarantee bad health. But vegetarians do seem to enjoy some health benefits, including lower blood cholesterol levels, lower blood pressure, and less risk of osteoporosis, gallstones, and diabetes. In the past, many child health experts expressed concern as to whether vegetarian diets were beneficial for *children*, but now most agree that a well-planned lacto-ovo- or lacto-vegetarian diet is compatible with normal growth and development.

Vegan diets are viewed with more concern. Researchers have found that vegan children tend to be shorter and lighter than other vegetarians or children who eat meat, though they fall within the normal range of growth. There have been a few horror stories of rickets, and vitamin B_{12} deficiencies.

Vegan food patterns are typically high in fiber and low in calories; it can be difficult for a small child to eat enough to satisfy her calorie requirements. Fiber can hinder the absorption of iron, calcium, and zinc. Inadequate protein, calcium, essential fatty acids, riboflavin, iron, zinc, vitamin D, or vitamin B_{12} all are potentially matters of concern in a vegan diet, especially if the child is a picky eater and rejects good sources of these nutrients.

It's quite simple to work out an adequate diet for a child who eats dairy products and eggs. Planning to meet the needs of the vegan child requires considerably more effort.

> **Meal Planning for Vegan Children**
>
> - Use soy milk or formula fortified with vitamins D and B$_{12}$.
> - Use cooked dried beans, nuts and nut butters, and seeds as meat alternates.
> - Tofu can be a good source of calcium, but only if it is made with calcium sulfate...check the label. Corn tortillas and greens like kale, bok choy, and collards are also high in calcium.
> - Serve foods rich in vitamin C at meals to enhance iron absorption.
> - Children may require more frequent meals and snacks because vegan meals tend to be filling but low in calories.
> - Consider serving eggs and dairy products to very young children or children who are picky eaters and not growing well.

For excellent discussions of vegetarian meal planning and delicious recipes, we highly recommend: *The New Laurel's Kitchen*, by Laurel Robertson, Carol Flinders, and Brian Ruppenthal. Berkekely, California: Ten Speed Press, 1986.

❏   ❏   ❏

Vitamin and Mineral Supplements

Over half of preschool- and school-age children receive multivitamin-mineral supplements. Often these children aren't the ones who could really benefit from them.[1]

Parents usually give vitamin and mineral supplements to their children because they feel the need for some insurance against the ups and downs of their children's appetites. Some are using these supplements as alternatives to conventional medical therapy for a variety of health problems. For some children supplements may be helpful, for others they are harmless but a waste of money, and for others they can cause significant problems:[60]

❏ It isn't necessarily true that if a little of a nutrient is good, more is better; some nutrients are toxic at high doses, and they may interfere with the body's ability to use other nutrients.

❏ Vitamin-mineral supplements can give parents a false sense of security about their children's diets; these supplements contain only a fraction of the many nutrients needed for health.

❏ Children can get the message that pills, not nutritious foods are necessary for growing into healthy adulthood.

❏ Children have mistaken vitamin or mineral supplements for candy and died from overdoses.

The American Academy of Pediatrics has determined that most children don't need vitamin or mineral supplements. Those who probably do are:[65]

- ❏ children whose diet is significantly limited because of such conditions as severe allergies, developmental delays, serious feeding problems, or poor appetite
- ❏ children living in neglectful or abusive situations
- ❏ children consuming a vegan diet
- ❏ pregnant teenagers

Parents who decide to give their children vitamin or mineral supplements should treat them as medications and keep them out of the reach of young children. Unless instructed otherwise by a physician, it's best to avoid giving a supplement that contains more than 100% of the RDA for any nutrient.[36]

APPENDIX C

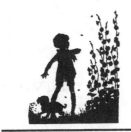

References

Chapter One —Introduction

1. National Education Association. *The Relationship Between Nutrition and Learning: A School Employee's Guide to Information and Action.* Washington, D.C.: National Education Association of the United States, 1989.

2. U.S. Department of Health and Human Services, Public Health Service. *The Surgeon General's Report on Nutrition and Health.* Washington, D.C.: U.S. Government Printing Office, 1988.

3. Satter, E. *How to Get Your Kid to Eat . . . But Not Too Much.* Palo Alto: Bull Publishing, 1987.

4. Sombke, L.: How our meals have changed. *USA Weekend,* November 11–13, 1988.

5. Satter, E. *How to Get Your Kid to Eat . . . But Not Too Much.*

6. Story, M. and Brown, J.E.: Do children instinctively know what to eat? The studies of Clara Davis revisited. *New England Journal of Medicine* 316(2): 103–106, 1987.

7. Satter, E. *How to Get Your Kid to Eat . . . But Not Too Much.*

Chapter Two—Feeding and Growth

1. Pipes, P.L.: Infant feeding and nutrition. In *Nutrition in Infancy and Childhood,* Fourth Edition. St. Louis: Times Mirror/Mosby College Publishing, 1989.

2. Beal, V.: The preschool years (one to six). In *Nutrition in the Life Span.* New York: John Wiley & Sons, 1980.

3. DeBruyne, L.K. and Rolfes, S.R.: Infants: a nurtured beginning. In *Life Cycle Nutrition: Conception Through Adolescence.* St. Paul: West Publishing Company, 1989.

4. Fomon, S.J.: Reflections on infant feeding in the 1970s and 1980s. *American Journal of Clinical Nutrition* 46: 171, 1987.

5. Nelms, B.C. and Mullins, R.G. *Growth and Development: A Primary Health Care Approach.* Englewood Cliffs, N.J.: Prentice-Hall, Inc., 1982.

6. Radbill, S.X.: Infant feeding through the ages. *Clinical Pediatrics* 20: 613, 1981.

7. Committee on Nutrition, American Academy of Pediatrics: The use of whole cow's milk in infancy. *Pediatrics* 72: 253, 1983.

8. Food and Nutrition Service. *Feeding Infants: A Guide for Use in the Child Care Food Program.* Washington, D.C.: U.S. Department of Agriculture, 1988.

9. Committee on Nutrition, American Academy of Pediatrics: Follow-up or weaning formulas. *Pediatrics* 83: 1067, 1989.

10. Satter, E. *Child of Mine: Feeding with Love and Good Sense.* Palo Alto: Bull Publishing Co., 1986.

11. Hagan, J.: Out of the jar or homemade: what's best for baby and when? *Environmental Nutrition* 13: 1, 6–7, 1990.

12. *Exchange Lists for Meal Planning.* The American Diabetes Association, Inc. and The American Dietetic Association. 1986.

13. Pipes, P.L.: Nutrition: growth and development. In *Nutrition in Infancy and Childhood,* Fourth Edition. St. Louis: Times Mirror/Mosby College Publishing, 1989.

14. DeBruyne, L.K. and Rolfes, S.R.: Focal point 3: dental health. In *Life Cycle Nutrition: Conception Through Adolescence.* St. Paul: West Publishing Company, 1989.

15. Pipes, P.L.: Between infancy and adolescence. In *Nutrition in Infancy and Childhood,* Fourth Edition. St. Louis: Times Mirror/Mosby College Publishing, 1989.

16. Satter, E. *How to Get Your Kid to Eat . . . But Not Too Much.* Palo Alto: Bull Publishing Company, 1987.

17. Morgan, K.J. and Zabik, M.E.: Amount and food sources of total sugar intake by children ages 5 to 12 years. *American Journal of Clinical Nutrition* 34: 404, 1981.

18. Gortmaker, S.L., Dietz, W.H., and Cheung, L.W.Y.: Inactivity, diet, and the fattening of America. *Journal of the American Dietetic Association* 90: 1247, 1990.

Chapter Three—Planning How and What to Feed Children

1. Satter, E: The feeding relationship. *Child of Mine: Feeding with Love and Good Sense.* Palo Alto: Bull Publishing Co., 1986.

2. U.S. Department of Agriculture, U.S. Department of Health and Human Services. *Nutrition and Your Health: Dietary Guidelines for Americans.* Washington, D.C.: U.S. Government Printing Office, 1990.

3. Pipes, P.L.: Infant feeding and nutrition. In *Nutrition in Infancy and Childhood.* Fourth Edition. St. Louis: Times Mirror/Mosby College Publishing, 1989.

4. Nutrition Division, Calgary Health Services. *Day Care Nutrition and Food Service Manual.* Calgary, Alberta: Calgary Health Services, 1988.

5. Child Care Food Program. *Simplified Buying Guide, 1987 Edition.* Sacramento: California State Department of Education, 1987.

Chapter Six—Running a Ship-Shape Kitchen

1. Bailey, Janet. *Keeping Food Fresh.* New York: Harper & Row, Publishers, 1989.

2. Satter, E.: Diarrhea. *Child of Mine: Feeding with Love and Good Sense.*

3. U.S. Department of Agriculture, Human Nutrition Information Service. *Shopping for Food and Making Meals in Minutes Using the Dietary Guidelines.* Washington, D.C.: U.S. Government Printing Office, 1989.

4. Blume, E.: Germ wars. Cleaning up our food. *Nutrition Action Healthletter* 13 (6): 1, 1986.

5. Miller, R.: Mother Nature's regulations on food safety. *FDA Consumer,* April 1988.

6. Blumenthal, D.: An unwanted souvenir . . . lead in ceramic ware. *FDA Consumer,* December 1989-January 1990.

7. Hillman, H. *Kitchen Science,* Revised Edition. Boston: Houghton Mifflin Company, 1989.

8. _____, *Sunset Microwave Cook Book.* Menlo Park, CA: Lane Publishing, 1981.

9. Farley, Dixie: Keeping up with the microwave revolution. *FDA Consumer,* March 1990.

10. Lefferts, Lisa Y. and Schmidt, Stephen: Microwaves: the heat is on. In *Nutrition Action Healthletter.* 17(1): January/February, 1990.

11. Large microwave ovens. In *Consumer Report.* 55(11), November 1990.

12. Microwave heating of infant formula and breast milk. In *Child Health Alert,* July 1990.

13. How safe is the microwave for kids? In *American Health: Fitness of Body and Mind.* 9(7): September, 1990.

14. How safe is the microwave for kids? In *American Health: Fitness of Body and Mind.*

Chapter Seven—Environmental Concerns

1. Smith, Kirk B.: Home Economics. In *The Green Lifestyle Handbook: 1001 Ways You Can Heal the Earth.* New York: Henry Holt & Co.,1990.

2. Earthworks Group and Pacific Gas & Electric. *30 Simple Energy Things You Can Do to Save the Earth.* 1990.

3. MacEachern, Diane. *Save Our Planet: 750 Everyday Ways You Can Help Clean Up the Earth.* New York: Dell Publishing, 1990.

4. MacEachern, Diane. *Save Our Planet: 750 Everyday Ways You Can Help Clean Up the Earth.*

5. MacEachern, Diane. *Save Our Planet: 750 Everyday Ways You Can Help Clean Up the Earth.*

6. Morris, David: A materials policy from the ground up. In *The Green Lifestyle Handbook: 1001 Ways You Can Heal the Earth.* New York: Henry Holt & Co., 1990.

7. Hadingham, Evan and Janet. *Garbage! Where It Comes From, Where It Goes.* New York: Simon and Schuster, Inc., 1990.

8. Kimbrell, Andrew C.: Environmental house cleaning. In *The Green Lifestyle Handbook: 1001 Ways You Can Heal the Earth*

9. Dadd, Debra Lynn. *The Nontoxic Home.* Los Angeles: Jeremy P. Tarcher, Inc., 1986

10. Dadd, Debra Lynn . *Nontoxic and Natural: How to Avoid Dangerous Everyday Products and Buy or Make Safe Ones.* Los Angeles: Jeremy P. Tarcher, Inc., 1984

11. Earthworks Group. *50 Simple Things Kids Can Do to Save the Earth.* Kansas City: Andrews and McMeel, 1990

12. Earthworks Group. *The Recycler's Handbook: Simple Thing You Can Do.* Berkeley: Earth Works Press, 1990

13. Elkington, J., Hailes, J., Hill, D. & Makower, J. *Going Green: A Kid's Handbook to Saving the Planet.* New York: The Penguin Group, 1990.

14. Heloise. *Heloise: Hints For A Healthy Planet.* New York: The Putnam Publishing Group, 1990.

15. Lamb, Marjorie. *2 Minutes a Day for a Greener Planet: Quick and Simple Things Americans Can Do to Save the Earth.* New York: Harper & Row, Publishers, Inc., 1990.

Appendix A—Nutrition Basics

1. Food and Nutrition Board, National Research Council; *Recommended Dietary Allowances.* Washington, DC; National Academy of Sciences, 1989.

2. U.S. Department of Agriculture, U.S. Department of Health and Human Services. *Nutrition and Your Health: Dietary Guidelines for Americans.* Washington, DC, 1990.

3. Christakis, G. (ed.). *Nutritional Assessment in Health Programs.* Washington, DC: American Public Health Association, Inc., 1973.

Appendix B—Special Topics

1. Pipes, P.: Nutritional needs of infants and children. In *Nutrition in Infancy and Childhood,* Fourth Edition. St. Louis: Times Mirror/Mosby College Publishing, 1989.

2. Levine, E.: Food allergies: cause for concern or over-diagnosed malady? *Environmental Nutrition* 12 (11): 1, 1989.

3. Cant, A.J.: Food allergy in childhood. *Human Nutrition: Applied Nutrition* 39A: 277, 1985.

4. Bock, S.A.: Prospective appraisal of complaints of adverse reactions to foods in children during the first 3 years of life. *Pediatrics* 79: 683, 1987.

5. Pipes, P.: Special concerns of dietary intake during infancy and childhood. In *Nutrition in Infancy and Childhood,* Fourth Edition.

6. Fomon, S.J.: Reflections on infant feeding in the 1970s and 1980s. *American Journal of Clinical Nutrition* 46: 171, 1987.

7. *The Relationship Between Nutrition and Learning: A School Employee's Guide to Information and Action.* Washington, D.C.: National Education Association, 1989.

8. Oski, F.A.: Iron deficiency—facts and fallacies. *Pediatric Clinics of North America* 32: 493, 1985.

9. Florentino, R.F. and Guirriec, R.M.: Prevalence of nutritional anemia in infancy and childhood with emphasis on developing countries. In Steckel, A., editor: *Iron Nutrition in Infancy and Childhood.* New York: Nestle, Vevey/Raven Press, 1984.

10. Satter, E.: Feeding the toddler. In *Child of Mine: Feeding with Love and Good Sense.* Palo Alto: Bull Publishing Company, 1986.

11. Harris, C.S., Baker, S.P., Smith, G.A., and Harris, R.M.: Childhood asphyxiation by food. A national analysis and overview. *Journal of the American Medical Association* 251: 2231, 1984.

12. Pipes, P.: Between infancy and childhood. In *Nutrition in Infancy and Childhood,* Fourth Edition.

13. Food and Nutrition Service. *Feeding Infants: A Guide for Use in the Child Care Food Program.* Washington, D.C.: U.S. Department of Agriculture, 1988.

14. Project Care for Children: *Childhood Emergencies—What to Do.* Palo Alto: Bull Publishing Company, 1987.

15. Rappaport, L.A. and Levine, M.D.: The prevention of constipation and encopresis: a developmental model and approach. *Pediatric Clinics of North America* 33: 859, 1986.

16. DeBruyne, L.K. and Rolfes, S.R.: Focal point 3: dental health. In *Life Cycle Nutrition: Conception Through Adolescence.* St. Paul: West Publishing Company, 1989.

17. Siminerio, L.M. and Betschart, J.: *Children with Diabetes.* Alexandria, VA: The American Diabetes Association, Inc., 1986.

18. Diet for cystic fibrosis. In *Manual of Clinical Dietetics.* Chicago: The American Dietetic Association, 1988.

19. Inborn errors of metabolism. In *Manual of Clinical Dietetics.* Chicago: The American Dietetic Association, 1988.

20. Satter, E.: Feeding the child with special needs. In *How to Get Your Kid to Eat . . . But Not Too Much.* Palo Alto: Bull Publishing Company, 1987.

21. Satter, E.: Diarrhea. In *Child of Mine: Feeding with Love and Good Sense.*

22. Committee on Nutrition, American Academy of Pediatrics: Use of oral fluid therapy and posttreatment feeding following enteritis in children in a developed country. *Pediatrics* 75: 358, 1985.

23. Nutritional management of diarrhea in childhood. In *Manual of Clinical Dietetics.* Chicago: The American Dietetic Association, 1988.

24. Cohen, S.A., Hendricks, K.M., Eastham, E.J., Mathis, R.K., and Walker, W.A.: Chronic nonspecific diarrhea, a complication of dietary fat restriction. *American Journal of Diseases in Childhood* 133: 490, 1979.

25. Green, H.L. and Ghishan, F.K.: Excessive fluid intake as a cause of chronic diarrhea in young children. *Journal of Pediatrics* 102: 836, 1983.

26. Hyams, J.S., Etienne, N.L., Leichtner, A.M., and Theuer, R.C.: Carbohydrate malabsorption following fruit juice ingestion in young children. *Pediatrics* 82: 64, 1988.

27. Hyams, J.S. and Leichtner, A.M.: Apple juice: an unappreciated cause of chronic diarrhea. *American Journal of Diseases in Childhood* 139: 503, 1985.

28. Lloyd-Still, J.D.: Chronic diarrhea of childhood and the misuse of elimination diets. *Journal of Pediatrics* 95: 10, 1979.

29. Satter, E.: Eating disorders. In *Child of Mine: Feeding with Love and Good Sense.*

30. Satter, E.: Eating disorders. In *How to Get Your Kid to Eat . . . But Not Too Much.*

31. Powers, D.E. and Moore, A.O.: *Food Medication Interactions.* Phoenix: F-M I Publishing, 1986.

32. Shapiro, L.R., Crawford, P.B., Clark, M.J., Pearson, D.J., Ray, J., and Huenemann, R.L.: Obesity prognosis: a longitudinal study of children from the age of 6 months to 9 years. *American Journal of Public Health* 74: 968, 1984.

33. Accounting for taste. *University of California, Berkeley, Wellness Letter* 7: 7, 1990.

34. Satter, E.: Nutritional tactics for preventing food fights. In *How to Get Your Kid to Eat . . . But Not Too Much.*

35. Committee on Nutrition, American Academy of Pediatrics: Practical significance of lactose intolerance in children: supplement. *Pediatrics* 86: 643, 1990.

36. Committee on Diet and Health, Food and Nutrition Board, National Research Council: Recommendations. In *Diet and Health: Implications for Reducing Chronic Disease Risk.* Washington, D.C.: National Academy Press, 1989.

37. Committee on Nutrition, American Academy of Pediatrics: Prudent life-style for children: dietary fat and cholesterol. *Pediatrics* 78: 521, 1986.

38. Pugliese, M.T., Weyman-Daum, M., Moses, N., and Lifshitz, F.: Parental health beliefs as a cause of nonorganic failure to thrive. *Pediatrics* 80: 175, 1987.

39. Lifshitz, F. and Moses, N.: Growth failure. A complication of dietary treatment of hypercholesterolemia. *American Journal of Diseases in Childhood* 143: 537, 1989.

40. Newman, W., Freedman, D.S. and Voors, A.W.: Relation of serum lipoprotein levels and systolic blood pressure to early atherosclerosis. *New England Journal of Medicine* 314: 138, 1986.

41. Gortmaker, S.L., Dietz, W.H., and Cheung, L.W.Y.: Inactivity, diet, and the fattening of America. *Journal of the American Dietetic Association* 90: 1247, 1990.

42. Peck, E.B. and Ullrich, H.D.: *Children and Weight: A Changing Perspective.* Berkeley: Nutrition Communications Associates, 1988.

43. Hermann, M.: EN speaks with obesity expert. *Environmental Nutrition* 13: 1, 1990.

44. Liebman, B.: Calories don't count . . . equally. *Nutrition Action Healthletter* 16 (1):8, 1989.

45. Satter, E.: Helping all you can to keep your child from being fat. In *How to Get Your Kid to Eat . . . But Not Too Much.*

46. Lefferts, L.: Pass the pesticides. *Nutrition Action Healthletter* 16 (3): 1, 1989.

47. Montgomery, A.: America's pesticide-permeated food. *Nutrition Action Healthletter* 14 (5): 1, 1987.

48. Ames, B: Dietary carcinogens and anticarcinogens. *Science,* 221: 1256, 1983.

49. Food and Nutrition Board, National Research Council: *Recommended Dietary Allowances.* Washington, D.C.: National Academy of Sciences, 1989.

50. *Sodium Scoreboard.* Washington, D.C.: Center for Science in the Public Interest.

51. Wrap-up: sodium. *University of California, Berkeley Wellness Letter,* 2(7): 4, 1986.

52. Pipes, P.: Nutrition and feeding of children with developmental delay and related problems. In *Nutrition in Infancy and Childhood,* Fourth Edition.

53. Whitney, E.N., Cataldo, C.B., and Rolfes, S.R.: Nutrition and behavior. In *Understanding Normal and Clinical Nutrition.* St. Paul: West Publishing Company, 1988.

54. Bachorowski, J., Newman, J.P., Nichols, S.L., Gans, D.A., Harper, A.E., and Taylor, S.L.: Sucrose and delinquency: behavioral assessment. *Pediatrics* 86: 244, 1990.

55. Kaplan, B.J., McNichol, J., Conte, R.A., and Moghadam, H.K.: Dietary replacement in preschool-aged hyperactive boys. *Pediatrics* 83: 7, 1989.

56. Sugar may jolt adrenaline in kids. *Environmental Nutrition* 13(7): 3, 1990.

57. Committee on Communications, American Academy of Pediatrics: Children, adolescents, and television. *Pediatrics* 85: 1119, 1990.

58. Trahms, C.: Factors that shape food patterns in young children. In *Nutrition in Infancy and Childhood,* Fourth Edition. St. Louis: Times Mirror/Mosby College Publishing, 1989.

59. Schmidt, S.: Hawking food to kids. *Nutrition Action Healthletter* 16(1): 1, 1989.

60. *Promoting Nutritional Health During the Preschool Years: Canadian Guidelines.* Network of the Federal/ Provincial/ Territorial Group on Nutrition and National Institute of Nutrition, 1989.

61. TV, kids' cholesterol linked. *San Francisco Chronicle,* November 14, 1990.

62. Satter, E.: The child who grows poorly. In *How to Get Your Kid to Eat . . . But Not Too Much.*

63. Trahms, C.: Vegetarian diets for children. In *Nutrition in Infancy and Childhood,* Fourth Edition. St. Louis: Times Mirror/Mosby College Publishing, 1989.

64. O'Connell, J.M., Dibley, M.J., Sierra, J., Wallace, B., Marks, J.S., and Yip, R.: Growth of vegetarian children: the Farm study. *Pediatrics* 84: 475, 1989.

65. Committee on Nutrition, American Academy of Pediatrics: Vitamin and mineral supplement needs of normal children in the United States. *Pediatrics* 66: 1015, 1980.

APPENDIX D

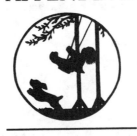

Resources

Publications

General Nutrition

Nutrition Action Healthletter
Center for Science in the Public Interest
Suite 300, 1875 Connecticut Avenue, N.W.
Washington, D.C. 20009-5728
$14.95/year
Reports on the latest nutrition research and consumer issues; includes great recipes.

University of California, Berkeley Wellness Letter
Wellness Letter Subscription Department
P.O. Box 420148
Palm Coast, Florida 32142
$20/year
"The newsletter of nutrition, fitness, and stress management"

Tufts University
Diet & Nutrition Letter
P.O. Box 57857
Boulder, CO 80322-7857
1-800-274-7581
Subscription $20 per year (12 issues)

Consumer Information Catalog Booklets
(When ordering free booklets, you must enclose $1.00 to help defray costs.) To order sales and free booklets, include check or money order payable to: Superintendent of Documents, and mail to:
R. Woods
Consumer Information Center-T
P.O. Box 100
Pueblo, Colorado 81002

Dietary Guidelines Booklets. Four colorful magazine-style booklets to help put the USDA/HHS Dietary Guidelines for Americans into everyday practice:

1. *"Eating Better When Eating Out"* How to compare calories and nutrients; with sample menu to help build food selection skills. 19 pp. (1989. USDA/HHS); Item # 123W. $1.50.

2. *"Making Bag Lunches, Snacks, and Desserts."* Ideas for creative hot and cold lunches; snack and dessert ideas with less fat and sugar. 31 pp. (1989. USDA/HHS); Item # 124W. $2.50.

3. *"Preparing Foods and Planning Menus."* Sample daily menus at two different calorie levels with recipes and tips for cutting down fat, sugars and sodium. 31 pp. (1989. USDA/HHS); Item # 125W. $2.50.

4. *"Shopping for Food and Making Meals in Minutes."* An aisle-by-aisle shopping guide to the supermarket; includes time saving recipes. 35 pp. (1989. USDA/HHS); Item #126W. $3.00.

Other booklets from Consumer Information Catalog:

"Eating for Life." How food choices can reduce your risk of developing cancer and heart diseases. Tips on buying and preparing food and eating out. 23 pp. (1988. NIH); Item #118W. $1.00.

"Nutritive Value of Foods." Listings for over 900 foods—calories, sodium, cholesterol and more. 72 pp. (1988. USDA); 120W. $2.75.

"Planning a Diet for a Healthy Heart." Learn how to reduce the risk of heart disease by cutting down on fat and cholesterol. 6 pp. (1989. FDA); Item #525W. Free.

"Food Additives." Explains why chemicals are added to foods and how this is regulated. 4 pp. (1987. FDA); Item #523W. Free.

Food News for Consumers. Up-to-date articles on food safety, health and nutrition, food concerns. Annual subscription/4 issues (USDA); Item #251W. $5.00.

Jane Brody's Nutrition Book by Jane Brody Toronto: Bantam Books, 1987

The New Laurel's Kitchen by, L. Robertson, C. Flinders, and, B. Ruppenthal. Berkeley: Ten Speed Press, 1986.

Child Nutrition

Child of Mine: Feeding With Love and Good Sense by Ellyn Satter, RD, MS, MSSW. Palo Alto: Bull Publishing Co.,1986.

How to Get Your Kid to Eat . . . But Not Too Much by Ellyn Satter RD, MS, MSSW. Palo Alto: Bull Publishing Co., 1987.

The Relationship Between Nutrition and Learning: A School Employees' Guide to Information and Action. National Education Association
Human and Civil Rights
1201 Sixteenth Street, N.W.
Washington, D.C., 20036
(800) 229-4200
Describes the importance of nutrition for optimum learning and what schools can do to ensure that all children have access to good nutrition.

Allergies

Allergy Products Directory
Prologue Publications
P.O. Box 640
Menlo Park, CA 94026.
Listings for food products and their sources.

"Tasty Rice Recipes for Those With Allergies"
Rice Council of America
P.O. Box 74021
Houston, TX 77274

"Gluten-Free Diet"
National Celiac-Sprue Society
5 Jeffrey Road
Wayland, MA 01778

"Delicious Milk-Free Recipes"
Loma Linda Foods
11503 Pierce Street
Riverside, CA 92515

Coping With Food Allergy by Claude A. Frazier, M.D. Revised Edition. New York: Times Books, 1985.
Good information on food allergies with extensive recipe section.

Caring and Cooking for the Allergic Child by Linda Thomas. New York: Sterling Publishing, 1980.

Diabetes

American Diabetes Association, Inc.
Diabetes Information Service Center
1660 Duke Street
Alexandria, VA 22314
(800)ADA-DISC
Also local affiliates.

Diabetes Mellitus—A Practical Handbook by Sue K. Milchovich, RN, BSN, CDE, and Barbara Dunn-Long, RD. Palo Alto: Bull Publishing Co., 1990.

Exchanges for All Occasions: Meeting the Challenge of Diabetes by Marion J. Franz, RD, MS. Minnesota: Diabetes Center, Inc., 1987. Diabetic exchange lists, recipes, and hints for managing events like illness, travel and children's parties.

Kids, Food, and Diabetes by Gloria Loring Chicago: Contemporary Books, Inc., 1986. Written by an actress and mother of a child with diabetes, this book is full of guidelines, recipes, and "coping hints" for dealing with diabetes.

Special Needs

"Feeding Young Children with Cleft Lip and Palate" (booklet, $1.50)
Minnesota Dietetic Association
1821 U. Avenue, Suite S-280
St. Paul, MN 55104

United Cerebral Palsy Associations, Inc.
66 East 34th Street
New York, NY 10016
(212) 481-6344

American Occupational Therapy Assoc., Inc.
1383 Piccard Drive
P.O. Box 1725
Rockville, MD 20850-4375

Mealtimes for Persons with Severe Handicaps by R. Perske, A. Clifton, B.M. McLean and J. Ishler Stein. Baltimore: Paul H. Brookes, 1986.
Managing the School-Age Child With a Chronic Health Condition, Georgianna Larson, RN, PNP, MPH, Editor.
Minnesota: DCI Publishing, 1988.

Food Safety

For Our Kids' Sake: How to Protect Your Child Against Pesticides in Food by Anne Witte Garland. San Francisco: Sierra Club Books, 1989.

FDA Consumer
Annual subscription (10 issues), $12.00 Item #252W Articles on safety of food, drugs, and cosmetics and their regulation by the Food and Drug Administration.

Food News for Consumers
Annual subscription (4 issues), $5.00 Item #251W.

To subscribe to *FDA Consumer* or *Food News for Consumers* make check or money order payable to Superintendent of Documents and send order to:
Consumer Information Center - T
P.O. Box 100
Pueblo, CO 81002

Cookbooks

Jane Brody's Good Food Book by Jane Brody Toronto: Bantam Books, 1987.
More than 350 healthful recipes and lots of good basic nutrition information.

The New Laurel's Kitchen by , L. Robertson, C. Flinders, and B. Ruppenthal.
Berkeley: Ten Speed Press, 1986.

Healthwise Quantity Cookbook by S.Turner, MPH, RD and V. Aronowitz, MPH, RD. Washington, D.C.: Center for Science in the Public Interest, 1990.

Cooking Light magazine.
P.O. Box 830549
Birmingham, AL 35282-9810

Microwave Diet Cookery by M. Cone & T. Snyder. New York: Simon and Schuster, 1988. How to use the microwave oven to prepare low-calorie, healthy meals.

Kitchen Lore

Keeping Food Fresh: How to Choose and Store Everything You Eat, by Janet Bailey. Revised Edition. New York: Harper & Row, Publishers. New York, 1989.This book contains fascinating information on selecting and storing foods and general tips for food safety.

Kitchen Science: A Guide to Knowing the How's and Why's for Fun and Success in the Kitchen. Revised Edition. Boston: Houghton Mifflin Company, 1989. For those who wonder— How do nonstick coatings work? Why does meat get tougher as it cooks? Why does red cabbage turn bluish purple when cooked?

Social and Environmental Concerns

Discovering the World: Empowering Children to Value Themselves, Others and the Earth. S. Hopkins and J. Winters, ed. Philadelphia, PA: New Society Publishers, 1990.

Anti-Bias Curriculum: Tools for Empowering Young Children by Louise Derman-Sparks and the A.B.C. Task Force. Washington, D.C.: National Association for the Education of Young Children, 1989. (companion video also available)

Food First Curriculum: An integrated curriculum for Grade 6 by Laurie Rubin. San Francisco, CA: Institute for Food and Development Policy, 1984.

Teaching and Learning in a Diverse World: Multicultural Education for Young Children by Patricia G. Ramsey. Available from Toys 'n Things Press; (800) 423-8309.

An Introductory Guide to Bilingual Bicultural/ Multicultural Education: Beyond Tacos, Eggrolls and Grits by Gloria Gomez. Dubuque: Kendall/Hunt Publishing Company, 1982.

Skipping Stones
Aprovecho Institute
80574 Hazelton Rd.
Cottage Grove, OR 97424; (503) 942-9434.
$15/year (quarterly).
A multi-ethnic international children's magazine.

50 Simple Things Kids Can Do to Save the Earth by The Earthworks Group. Kansas City: Andrews and McMeel, 1990.

Children's Book Press
1461 Ninth Avenue
San Francisco, CA 94122
(415) 664-8500
A non-profit children's book publisher, specializing in multicultural children's literature.

Mothers and Others for a Livable Planet.
Natural Resources Defense Council
40 West 20th Street.
New York, NY 10011
(212) 727-2700
A special project dedicated to environmental problems that especially affect children. *TLC,* its newsletter, has a pull-out section for children.

Kids for Saving Earth
P.O. Box 47247
Plymouth, MN 55447-0247
(612) 525-0002
International membership organization for kids who pledge to "be a defender of my planet." Members receive certificate, resources, guidebook and more.

Garbage! Where It Comes From, Where It Goes by Evan & Janet Hadingham. New York: Simon and Schuster, Inc., 1990.

Going Green: A Kid's Handbook to Saving the Planet by J.Elkington, J. Hailes, D. Hill, and J. Makower. New York: Puffin Books, 1990.

Shopping for a Better World: The Quick and Easy Guide to Socially Responsible Supermarket Shopping
Council on Economic Priorities
30 Irving Place
New York, NY 10003-9990
(800) 822-6435
Provides the information necessary for consumers to select products made by companies whose policies and practices they support.

The Consumer Guide to Home Energy Savings
American Council for an Energy Efficient Economy
1001 Connecticut Avenue, NW, #535
Washington, DC 20036
(202) 429-8873
$6.95

Garbage: The Practical Journal for the Environment
P.O. Box 51647
Boulder, CO 80321-1647
An excellent resource for home waste-reduction.

Nutrition Activities with Kids

Creative Food Experiences for Children by Mary T. Goodwin and G. Pollen. Revised Edition. Washington, D.C.: Center for Science in the Public Interest, 1980. A classic guide to teaching children aged 3 to 10 about good nutrition.

Eat, Think, and Be Healthy! by Paula K. Zeller and M. Jacobsen, Ph.D. Washington, D.C.: Center for Science in the Public Interest, 1987. Nutrition activities for kids grade 3-6. Includes recipes for foods kids can make. Handouts. Basic nutrition, smart consumerism.

I Love Animals and Broccoli by Debra Wasserman and Charles Stahler. Baltimore: 1985.
The Vegetarian Resource Group
P.O. Box 1463, Baltimore MD 21203. $5.00.
Healthy eating, caring about animals, world hunger.

Cooking With Kids

Cook and Learn: Pictorial Single Portion Recipes by Beverly Veitch and Thelma Harms. Menlo Park: Addison-Wesley Publishing Company, 1981.

Kid's Cooking: A Very Slightly Messy Manual by the Editors of Klutz Press. Palo Alto: Klutz Press, 1987.

"Easy Menu Ethnic Cookbooks."
>   *Cooking the African Way*
>   *Cooking the Caribbean Way*
>   *Cooking the Chinese Way*
>   *Cooking the English Way*
>   *Cooking the French Way*
>   *Cooking the German Way*
>   *Cooking the Greek Way*
>   *Cooking the Hungarian Way*
>   *Cooking the Indian Way*
>   *Cooking the Israeli Way*
>   *Cooking the Italian Way*
>   *Cooking the Japanese Way*
>   *Cooking the Korean Way*
>   *Cooking the Lebanese Way*
>   *Cooking the Mexican Way*
>   *Cooking the Norwegian Way*
>   *Cooking the Polish Way*
>   *Cooking the Russian Way*
>   *Cooking the Spanish Way*
>   *Cooking the Thai Way*
>   *Cooking the Vietnamese Way*
>   —Lerner Publications
>   Company, Minneapolis

Miscellaneous Books

NAEYC Early Childhood Resources Catalog
1834 Connecticut Avenue, N.W.
Washington, D.C., 20009-5786
(800) 424-2460
Outstanding books, pamphlets, posters, etc., for early childhood educators from the National Association for the Education of Young Children.

Toys 'n Things Press: Resources for the Early Childhood Professional
A division of Resources for Child Caring
450 North Syndicate, Suite 5
St. Paul, MN 55104
(800) 423-8309
Excellent books and other learning materials for adults and children.

Supplies

Earth-Friendly Products

Seventh Generation, Products for a Healthy
Planet
Colchester, VT 05446-1672
(800) 441-2538
Energy-saving devices, ecological household
cleaners, recycling supplies. Catalog
includes lots of tips.

Co-op America Catalog
2100 M Street, Suite 403
Washington, DC 20063
(202) 223-1881
Ecological products, energy-saving devices,
etc.

Ecco Bella, The Environmental Store
6 Provost Square, Suite 602
Caldwell, NJ 07006
(800) 888-5320
Non-animal tested, bio-degradable products.

EcoSource, Products for a Safer, Cleaner
World
9051 Mill Station Rd.
Sebastopol, CA 95472
(800) 688-8345

Gardener's Supply
128 Intervale Road
Burlington, VT 05401
(802) 863-1700
Chemical-free pest control supplies,
composting equipment, etc.

Specialty Foods

Ener-G-Foods, Inc.
5960 - 1st Avenue S.
P.O. Box 84487
Seattle, WA 98124-5787
(800) 331-5222
Food products for gluten-free, wheat-free,
milk-free, soy-free, and corn-free diets.
Recipes also available.

Fearn Natural Foods
4520 James Place
Melrose Park, IL 60160
Baking mixes for allergy diets; found in most
health-food stores.

Loma Linda Foods
11503 Pierce Street
Riverside, CA 92515
A variety of food products for allergy diets.

Learning Materials and Toys

Good Food Puppets. Seven colorful
puppets—Milk, Chicken, Fish, Apple, Carrot,
Bread, SuperBean: $49.98/set. Good Food
Puppets Puppetry Book with scripts, lessons,
songs, etc.: $12.98/book. Complete set: $59.98.
To order, add 15% postage and handling fee.
Yummy Designs, P.O. Box 1851-D, Walla
Walla, WA 99362; (509)525-2072

Lingo, bingo-type game which familiarizes
children with foods around the world in three
languages (for 3–10 year olds).
UNICEF
1 Children's Boulevard, P.O. 182233
Chattanooga, TN 37422
(800) For-Kids

HearthSong
P.O. Box B
Sebastopol, CA 95473-0601
(800) 325-2502
Catalog of wonderful toys, crafts, books,
games, etc.

Animal Town
P.O. Box 485
Healdsburg, CA 95448
(800) 445-8642
Catalog of nature games and books,
cooperative games, posters, toys and much
more. Beautiful!

Music for Little People
P.O. Box 1460, 1144 Redway Drive
Redway CA 95560
(800) 346-4445
Children's audio and video tapes, musical
instruments. Materials which emphasize
multi-cultural, social and environmental
awareness.

Lakeshore® Learning Materials
2695 E. Dominguez Street. P.O. Box 6261
Carson, CA 90749
(800) 421-5354
Play foods (includes foods from various cultures), kitchen equipment, child-sized furniture; supplies for classroom cooking projects, etc.

Fisher-Price®
East Aurora, New York 14052
Super Mart Super Cart shopping cart comes with play money and groceries; Magic Scan Checkout Counter and other Fun with Food™ toys.

Miscellaneous

Fat Finder®
Vitaerobics
41-905 Boardwalk, Suite B
Palm Desert, CA 92260-5141
4 1/2-inch diameter wheel for quickly and accurately determining percentage of fat calories in foods. (16-inch demonstration model also available.) $5.45/$7.45 with 60-page book.

Lead Alert Kit
Francon Enterprises, Inc.
P.O. Box 300321, Seattle, WA 98103
(800) 359-9000
Tests pottery, toys, metalware, and decorated glassware for leaching of lead. $29.95 + $3.50 shipping

Table Manners for Everyday Use by Handy Vision. A humorous instructional video that can be enjoyed by both children and adults. Available from Sybervision Systems, Inc. (800) 678-0887

National Dairy Council®
Order Department*
6300 North River Road
Rosemont, IL 60018-4233
(708) 696-1860, Ext. 220
Curriculum packages for children, preschool through high school, and other consumer materials; some available in Spanish.
*Or check your telephone directory for a local Dairy Council® affiliate near you.

American Heart Association
44 East 23rd Street
New York, NY 10010
Check your telephone directory for a local AHA affiliate. A variety of educational materials are available, including schoolsite health promotion curricula.

The Vegetarian Resource Group
P.O. Box 1463
Baltimore, MD 21203
(301) 366-VEGE
Many free or low-cost teaching materials about vegetarianism, suitable for preschoolers through teens. Send for a resource list.

Community Resources and Organizations

Who to Ask for General Information

Local agencies:

- City, county, or state health department
- Cooperative Extension Service
- Women, Infants, and Children (WIC) supplemental food program
- Universities with programs in nutrition, dietetics, or food service management
- Child Care Food Program
- Affiliates of the American Heart Association, American Diabetes Association, American Cancer Society, or Dairy Council®

Consumer Information/Baby Food:

- Beech-Nut   (800) 523-6633
- Earth's Best   (800) 442-422
- Gerber   (800) 443-7237
- Heinz   (800) USA-BABY
- Simply Pure   (800) 426-7873

Food Safety Questions

Food and Drug Administration
Office of Consumer Affairs HFE-88
5600 Fishers Lane
Rockville, MD 20857
(301) 443-3170

USDA Meat and Poultry Hotline
USDA-FSIS, Room 1165-S
Washington, D.C. 20250
(800) 535-4555
(10 a.m. – 4 p.m. weekdays)

EPA Safe Drinking Water Hotline
(800) 426-4791
(202) 382-5533 in Washington, D.C.

Help for Children with Handicapping Conditions

- nutritionists in state and local health departments
- pediatric nutritionists, occupational therapists, and physical therapists in programs serving children with special needs, e.g., genetics treatment centers, diagnostic evaluation centers, and hospitals affiliated with a medical school

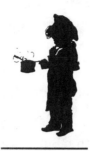

Recipe Index

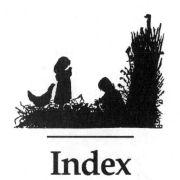

Index